Antonio Ja

Tantric Massage, the Complete Guide

A Journey Along The Path Of Ecstasy

Want to connect with Antonio Jaimez directly and be among the first to know about his latest releases and discover the works he is secretly working on? Join the exclusive members-only Facebook community and become part of a direct contact group with Antonio Jaimez. You will be able to leave your comments and proposals to improve his works and they will be heard. You will be able to interact with the community and you will also receive free content and exclusive promotions that Antonio will kindly share with his members.

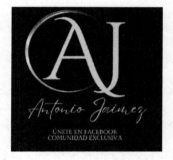

Click on this link to access the private Facebook group:

www.facebook.com/groups/antoniojaimezoficial/

Or scan the following QR code:

Preface: The Awakening: The Importance of Connection

Preface

Welcome dear reader! Your presence here is celebrated with joy and gratitude. I am Antonio Jaimez, your guide in this fascinating expedition you are about to begin. I am immensely honored that you have chosen this book as your companion on your journey of discovery and personal growth.

Your choice is a reflection of your wisdom and willingness to grow. You have demonstrated a valuable openness to new knowledge and experiences, a desire to discover the depths of your being and to connect with others on a deeper and more meaningful level. Let me congratulate you on this wise choice.

Throughout my life, I have been fortunate to learn and teach the practices and principles of tantric massage. It has been a passion, a vocation, a way of life. Through years of practice and teaching, I have seen and experienced firsthand the transformation it can bring into our lives. Now, I am pleased to be able to share that wisdom with you.

I consider myself a traveler and a perpetual learner on this path of ecstasy. Over the years, I have come to realize that authenticity, respect and compassion are the cornerstones for creating a safe and sacred space for the exploration of our divine essence. On every page of this book, you will find that essence.

We will begin this journey by diving into the ancient origins of tantric massage and the relevance of these practices today. Then, we will explore the magic and power of touch, senses and breath as pathways to awareness and connection. As we move forward, you will learn about the chakras, kundalini energy and how these concepts can enrich your tantric massage experience. Through this exploration, I invite you to open yourself to new perspectives, question cultural norms and cultivate a deeper relationship with yourself and others.

I know that as you continue reading this book, you will find tools and practices to connect with your sexual energy and transform it into a powerful vehicle for healing, creativity and spiritual growth. This book is designed not only to be read, but to be lived. I encourage you to practice, explore and immerse yourself in the experiences as you go along.

In addition to the knowledge and techniques, you will find in these pages a world of emotional benefits. Tantric massage can help you release emotional blockages, heal past wounds and cultivate greater acceptance and love for yourself. This path can be a path of liberation, empowerment and joy.

However, like any journey, there may be moments of uncertainty or challenge. If you encounter them, I invite you to persevere, to keep faith in your path and trust in the process. Always remember that you are not alone on this journey. I am here with you, supporting you

Chapter 1: The Origin of Tantric Massage: Ancient Practices Revisited

The most important journey you will ever undertake is the one that takes you from the outside to the inside, from the known to the unknown, from the routine to the mysterious. Are you ready to embark on such a journey? If you are reading these words, the answer is probably a resounding "yes". But have you ever wondered how the practice you are about to explore came about? How did the ancient wisdom of tantric massage find its place in contemporary society? And why is it so relevant today?

To fully understand tantric massage and its transformative power, it is essential to travel back in time, to its roots, to the origin of wisdom that has withstood the test of time and the storms of change. Here you will find the keys that will unlock your path to greater awareness, deeper connection and a life of fulfillment and ecstasy.

Tantric massage is neither a fad nor a modern invention. Its roots lie in ancient India, more than 5000 years ago, at a time when Indian sages codified a worldview that saw pleasure and spirituality as two sides of the same coin. Amazing, isn't it? In a world where duality seems to be the norm, where pleasure and spirituality are often seen as opposites, can you imagine how revolutionary this concept must have been? And what if I told you that this ancient wisdom still has the power to transform your life today?

But what exactly is tantric massage? Is it just an exotic form of massage, or is it something more? If you've ever heard the word "Tantra," you've probably been introduced to it as a way to prolong sexual pleasure or intensify intimacy in a couple's relationship. And, while these are part of the truth, they are not the whole truth.

Tantric massage is much more than a technique, it is a way of life, a philosophy, a path to ecstasy and liberation. But what exactly does that mean, and how can a "simple" massage be a path to ecstasy and liberation? These are profound questions, requiring careful and thoughtful exploration.

Tantra is a spiritual path that honors and celebrates sexual energy as a powerful and sacred force of life, creation and connection. This energy, when awakened and channeled correctly, is believed to have the potential to transform us, heal us and connect us to our divine essence.

Tantric massage is one of the most practical and accessible ways to explore this ancient philosophy. It combines breathing, meditation and massage techniques to awaken and channel sexual energy, fostering a deep connection with oneself and others.

But, make no mistake, it is not an easy task. It is not something that can be mastered overnight. It is a journey, a path, a pilgrimage to the very essence of who you are. And every journey, dear reader, requires courage, openness and patience. As the famous author and spiritual teacher Eckhart Tolle said in his book "The Power of Now" (1997), "Patience is not passive resignation, nor a renunciation of action; acting with awareness of being is its essence."

Ancient India, where Tantra flourished, was a land of contrasts and convergences. In the midst of this diversity, Tantra emerged as a revolutionary voice, challenging rigid structures and social norms. It advocated total acceptance of life in all its manifestations - the light and the dark, the sacred and the mundane, pleasure and pain.

And why do I mention all this? Well, because it is crucial to understand that the tantric massage we know today did not arise in a vacuum. It is the product of thousands of years of accumulated wisdom, of a tradition that has evolved and adapted through the ages and cultures.

But, although Tantric massage has its roots in ancient India, it is not limited to this culture. In fact, in its evolution, Tantra and its practices, including massage, have drawn from many sources and have been adapted to different cultures and times. As Professor and Tantra expert David Gordon White points out in his book "Enlightened Tantra" (2003), Tantra is "a product of synthesis and assimilation, a combination of elements from different traditions and cultures".

Therefore, the tantric massage we know today is as much a product of antiquity as it is of the present, a synthesis of ancient and modern wisdoms, a fusion of the Eastern and the Western. And this is precisely what makes it so relevant today.

And this is where you come into play. By opening this book, by embarking on this journey, you become part of this living history. You join an ancient tradition, you become an explorer of consciousness, an alchemist of ecstasy.

But what does all this mean for you, here and now? How can tantric massage enrich your life, here and now? How can it help you navigate the challenges of modern life, connect more deeply with yourself and others, live a life of greater fulfillment and ecstasy? These are the questions we will explore in the following pages. So, dear reader, I invite you to keep reading, keep exploring, keep opening yourself to the possibilities this book has to offer. Are you ready to continue the journey? Are you ready to delve even deeper into the fascinating world of tantric massage?

Here is a concrete example to help you visualize it better. Imagine you are in a beautiful garden filled with lush flowers and vibrant colors. The air is fresh and the sunlight filters through the leaves, creating a mosaic of shadows and dancing lights. You sit on a smooth stone and begin to feel life all around you: the buzzing of bees, the chirping of birds, the gentle rustle of leaves.

Do you notice how that sensory experience brings a sense of wholeness and presence? How, for a moment, all your problems and worries seem to dissolve into this here and now?

This is a glimpse of what tantric massage can offer you. But instead of being the spectator, you are both the garden and the gardener. You are the creator of your own ecstasy, the artisan of your own experience.

Tantric massage invites you to take the reins of your sensory life, to throw off the chains of routine and immerse yourself in the wonderful universe of sensations that dwells in your own body. And this is not a journey you should make alone.

Through tantric massage, you can learn to connect deeply with your partner, to communicate beyond words, to create together a space of intimacy, respect and shared ecstasy.

The well-known writer and teacher of Tantra, Margot Anand, in her work "The Art of Sexual Ecstasy: A Practical Manual on Tantric Love and Sex" (1995), tells us: "Tantra teaches us to accept our body, our needs and emotions, as sacred, to celebrate the dance of life and to touch others with awareness and respect".

Following this line of thought, tantric massage can be a wonderful tool to improve our relationships, to learn to give and receive love in a fuller and more conscious way.

Now, if you're feeling a little overwhelmed by all this, don't worry. We are here to explore together, step by step, on this journey of discovery and transformation. And, although it may seem like a long and challenging road, I assure you that every step is worth it. Each moment of presence, each conscious touch, each deep breath, brings you a little closer to yourself, to your essence, to your potential for love and ecstasy.

So, dear reader, I invite you to keep reading, to keep exploring, to keep growing. I promise you it will be a journey you will not forget. Are you ready to continue? Are you ready to dive deeper into the heart of tantric massage?

Are you ready to dive deeper into the heart of tantric massage? The answer to that question may seem simple, but in reality it has many layers. The choice to embark on this journey is not just a conscious decision, but a call from the heart, a whisper from the soul.

Beyond the techniques and practices, beyond the ancient scriptures and mysterious rituals, tantric massage is, in its essence, an invitation to love. To a love that expands beyond the limitations of the ego and merges with the whole. To a love that does not seek to possess, but to liberate. To a love that is not taken for granted, but cultivated with every breath, with every touch, with every heartbeat.

We are living at a time in history when the thirst for authentic connection, for deep intimacy, for genuine ecstasy, has never been greater. And tantric massage, with its focus on presence, awareness and connection, has the potential to answer this thirst, to provide an oasis in the desert of modern disconnection.

It doesn't matter if you are new to the world of tantra, if you have had previous experience with tantric massage, or if you are simply intrigued by what these pages can reveal to you. We are all here for a reason. We are all on this journey together. And together, we can explore, discover and transform.

Following in the footsteps of great masters of Tantra such as Osho, who in "Tantra: The Supreme Understanding" (1975) stated that "Tantra is the science of transforming ordinary lovers into soul mates. And that is the greatness of Tantra. It can transform all the energy of lust into love and prayer", we are invited to take our experiences of pleasure and connection to a whole new level.

We have already taken a look at the origin and philosophy of tantric massage. We have begun to discover how tantric massage can enrich our lives, enhance our relationships and unleash our potential for love and ecstasy.

But this, dear reader, is only the beginning. In the next chapter, "The Alchemy of Touch: From Skin to Soul," we will explore the importance of physical connection, the healing power of touch, and how we can use our hands not only to give pleasure, but to communicate love, respect and understanding.

Because on the path of tantric massage, every touch is a word, every caress is a phrase, and every encounter is a poem written in the language of the heart. I invite you to follow me on this journey, to open your mind and your heart, to discover your own path to ecstasy. Are you ready?

Chapter 2: The Alchemy of Touch: From Skin to Soul

Imagine that your hands are two powerful alchemists. These diligent magicians have the power to transform the ordinary into the extraordinary, to turn lead into gold. In the universe of skin, your hands have the ability to turn simple touch into a deep, spiritual connection. But what does this really mean, how can touch, something we see as merely physical, become a window to the soul?

I'm sure you can recall a time when someone's touch meant much more than mere physical contact. Perhaps it was a hug from a loved one after a long time apart, your partner's hand intertwined with yours in a moment of stillness, or even the casual brush of a friend that made you feel seen and understood. Touch has a language of its own, a language that speaks directly to the soul, crossing the barriers of verbal language and rationality.

This is the wonderful mystery of the alchemy of touch, the transformation of skin into soul, of touch into connection. But why is this alchemy of touch important, especially in the context of tantric massage?

Let me ask you a question, dear reader. Do you remember the last time you felt truly connected to someone, when you felt that all barriers were broken down and only the pure essence of each other remained? Do you remember how that felt in your body, on your skin?

Tantric massage, in its essence, seeks to cultivate and deepen this connection through conscious and loving touch. By connecting with our skin, the largest and one of the most sensitive organs of the human body, we open ourselves to a world of sensations and experiences that can take us beyond the limitations of our mind and emotions.

That's right, beloved reader, the skin is not simply a barrier that protects our body from the outside world. It is a boundary, a meeting point between self and other, between inner and outer. And when we touch and are touched with presence and love, this boundary can become a bridge, a portal to a deeper understanding of ourselves and others.

Throughout this chapter, we will embark on a deep and fascinating exploration of the alchemy of touch. We will discover together how touch can become a tool for healing, connection and awakening, and how tantric massage, with its focus on conscious, loving touch, can transform our experience of pleasure, love and intimacy. And remember, dear reader, this journey is as much yours as it is mine. So I invite you to explore, feel and open yourself to the wonderful possibilities this journey has to offer. Are you ready to begin?

The beauty of touch lies in its universality, you know, how a simple touch can communicate a multitude of emotions: love, compassion, comfort, desire, and so much more. But what if I told you that there is more to touch than what we might initially perceive? What if we explored touch not only as a means of physical communication, but also as a language of our soul?

To understand the true alchemy of touch, we must take a look at the teachings of neurobiology. As Candace Pert said in her groundbreaking book, "Molecules of Emotion" (1997), our body is literally our subconscious mind. Our emotions, thoughts and feelings are translated into chemical responses in our body, and these responses are perceived and felt through our sensory system. And among all our senses, touch is the most fundamental. Have you ever wondered why a hug can calm you down when you are sad, or why the touch of a beloved hand can make your heart beat faster?

All this is because touch, in its essence, is a holistic experience. It involves not only the skin and nerve endings, but also our emotions, our memory and our soul. Every touch is a symphony of sensations and emotions that speaks to us in a language deeper and more primordial than words.

To explain further, let us recall the teachings of Ashley Montagu in her work "Touching: The Human Significance of the Skin" (1971). Montagu proposed that the skin, with its millions of sensitive nerve endings, is a vehicle for love and connection. Through the skin, we connect with the outside world and communicate our inner needs and emotions. It is through the skin that we experience love, affection and intimacy.

Now, think of a tantric massage. Imagine two bodies intertwined in a sacred dance of touch and caress, of giving and receiving. In this space, touch is not just a means of transmitting physical pleasure. It is a way to express love, respect and reverence. It is a language that speaks to the heart and soul, that weaves a connection beyond the physical body. A tantric massage, when given and received with full awareness and love, can be a transformative experience, one that opens doors to greater connection, greater intimacy and, ultimately, greater understanding of self and other.

And perhaps now you are wondering, dear reader, how can you cultivate this alchemy of touch in your life? How can you transform your skin into a portal to your soul? Well, let me let you in on a secret: it all starts with presence and awareness. It all starts with conscious touch.

Have you ever found yourself completely absorbed in the simple act of touching something? Perhaps it was the soft, cozy texture of your favorite blanket, the roughness of a tree bark, or the liquid coolness of a bubbling brook? If so, my friend, then you have experienced the transformative power of a conscious touch.

Mindful touch is a state of mindfulness in which you are fully present in the act of touching and being touched. It is not an abstract concept, it is a tangible practice that you can integrate into your daily life, and tantric massage is a beautiful platform to explore and cultivate this mindful touch.

I am reminded of Michael Reed Gach's wisdom in Acupressure's Potent Points (1990) when he reminds us that "awareness is healing". In mindful touch, mindfulness and intention are key. It is not just about moving the hands, but about feeling, tuning in, being present with each touch and caress. When you touch with awareness, each touch becomes a meditation, an opportunity to deepen the connection with oneself and with the other.

Think of it this way: when you give a tantric massage, your hands become an instrument of your consciousness. You feel your partner's skin, their warmth, their texture, the contours of their muscles and bones. You feel their reactions, the way their body moves and responds to your touch. And in doing so, you become a conscious witness to their experience, an active participant in their journey toward greater bodily and spiritual awareness.

On the other hand, when you receive a tantric massage, your skin becomes a landscape of sensations. You open yourself to the experience of being touched, allowing yourself to receive love, care and pleasure. You surrender to the present, allowing yourself to feel every touch, every caress, every pressure. And in doing so, you connect more deeply with yourself, your body, your heart and your soul.

Now, imagine if you could bring this awareness of touch into every aspect of your life. Imagine that every hug is a celebration of connection, that every touch is an expression of love, that every touch is a poem written on the skin. In this world, skin is not just a sensory organ, but a portal to a deeper level of awareness and connection. In this world, every touch is an alchemy of love.

Do you feel ready to embark on this journey, my friend? Are you ready to explore the vast universe of sensations that dwells beneath your skin? Then join me, because this is just the beginning. In the following pages, we will delve deeper into the art and science of mindful touch, exploring its role in the practice of tantric massage and discovering how you can incorporate it into your daily life.

Like a gentle summer breeze gliding through a silk curtain, the essence of mindful touch is something you can only fully experience when you surrender to it, and not just in the context of tantric massage, but in every interaction you have with the tangible world.

Likewise, consider for a moment the words of Dacher Keltner in "Born to Be Good: The Science of a Meaningful Life" (2009), when he states that "touch is the primordial language of compassion". This concept is a cornerstone of tantric massage. Mindful touch, filled with intention and empathy, becomes a language we can use to express the ineffable, to convey love and acceptance, to provide comfort and relief, to establish a deep and meaningful connection with others.

As you reflect on what we have explored in this chapter, I invite you to meditate on the importance of this language of touch in your own life. How can you apply these principles of mindfulness and connection to the way you touch yourself, your partner, your loved ones, even the objects and nature around you? How can your life experience change when you commit to touching and being touched with full awareness and love?

And you know what? This is just the beginning. We are in the first steps of an incredibly exciting journey. In our next chapter, "Rediscovering Your Five Senses: The Portal to the Present," I invite you to delve even deeper into this wonderful exploration of the senses. We will go beyond the mere act of touch to explore how our five senses can be portals to deeper awareness and greater awakening.

Each of our senses offers us a unique way of interacting with the world, and by learning to use them more fully and with greater presence, we can enrich our experience of life in truly transformative ways. So, are you ready to embark on this sensory journey, my friend? Are you ready to discover the hidden secrets that await in the realm of the senses? Are you ready to explore the true alchemy of touch, not only in the realm of the skin, but also in the infinite garden of your soul?

Because that is the wonderful journey that awaits you in the next chapter. And believe me, it will be a life-changing experience, as each new discovery, each moment of enlightenment, will bring you one step closer to the essence of who you really are. So come, walk with me, because this journey to the heart of tantric massage is a journey to the heart of yourself.

Chapter 3: Rediscovering Your Five Senses: The Portal to the Present

There is an old Chinese proverb that says: "He who knows that he does not know, knows". Sound familiar? It may sound like a bit of a riddle, but it actually holds great wisdom. What it is trying to convey is that recognizing our ignorance is the first step towards wisdom. And in the context of our journey towards exploring tantric massage, this notion is especially pertinent.

Because, my friend, there's a good chance that, up until now, you've been living your life with a kind of blindfold on. It's not your fault. We live in a society that trains us to live in our heads, to focus on our thoughts and the future or the past, rather than the present.

I ask you a question, and it is important that you take a moment to reflect: When was the last time you really savored the food you were eating? Or paused to inhale the scent of a flower or the smell of wet earth after the rain? When was the last time you touched something, not out of necessity, but simply to enjoy the feel of its texture under your fingers?

If you can't remember, don't worry. You are not alone in this. Most of us are so disconnected from our senses, so caught up in our thoughts and worries, that we have forgotten how to be truly present in our bodies and in the world around us. And it is here, in this forgetfulness, that the importance of our five senses lies.

Our senses are the gateway to the present. They are the way we interact with the tangible world. Every time we savor a bite of food, smell the scent of a flower, feel the touch of the wind on our skin, hear a bird singing or contemplate a beautiful sunset, we are anchored in the here and now.

And why is it important to be present, you might ask? Well, presence is the very essence of tantric massage and, in fact, of any spiritual or consciousness practice. When we are present, we are fully engaged with the experience we are having. We are not thinking about what happened yesterday or what we have to do tomorrow. We are here, in this moment, living fully every second of our lives.

And the magic of presence is that, when we are fully present, we begin to notice things that were previously unnoticed. We discover beauty in unexpected places. We feel gratitude for the simplest things. We realize that each moment is a precious and ephemeral gift that will never be repeated in the same way.

So I invite you to join me on this journey to rediscover your five senses. To learn to see, hear, smell, taste and touch with new awareness. To open the doors of perception and live each moment to the fullest. I assure you it is an adventure that will change your life.

Now, let me take your imagination to an ancient forest, full of majestic, towering trees, with a great carpet of crunching leaves beneath your feet. Imagine closing your eyes and giving yourself permission to be fully present in this imaginary space. Can you feel the fresh air on your face? Can you hear the crunching of leaves under your feet, the wind blowing through the branches of the trees, the song of a bird in the distance? Can you smell the scent of damp earth and decaying leaves?

This simple visualization practice helps us understand how powerful our senses can be when we really take a moment to tune into them. You've noticed how you've felt more present, more alive, more connected to the world around you. This is just a glimpse of the transformation you can experience by rediscovering your five senses.

But you don't have to take my word for it. There are many other experts in the field of consciousness and spirituality who talk about the importance of being present and connected to our senses. For example, in his book "The Power of Now" (1997), Eckhart Tolle emphasizes the importance of living in the present moment and describes how our senses are the gateway to this awareness.

Also Jon Kabat-Zinn, in his book "Living Fully through Crises" (1990), introduces the practice of "mindfulness," which is basically a form of meditation that involves paying full attention to our experiences in the present moment, and yes, you guessed it, this includes paying attention to our senses.

These authors, and many others, have dedicated their lives to studying and teaching about the importance of living in the present moment and how our senses are an essential tool for this. But, despite all the words and studies, the only way to truly understand the power of our senses is to experience it for yourself.

So I invite you to take a short pause in your reading. Close your eyes and inhale deeply, filling your lungs with air until you can't take any more, and then exhale slowly. Repeat this several times and then do a quick scan of your senses. What do you hear? What do you smell? What do you feel on your skin? Is there a taste in your mouth?

You may be surprised at how much you can perceive when you really take the time to tune into your senses. And remember, this is just the beginning. Over the course of this chapter, we will explore each of our senses in greater depth and learn how we can use them to enhance our tantric massage practice and to live a fuller, more conscious life. Are you ready to continue on this fascinating journey?

Well, here we are, immersed in the rich texture of our senses, ready to explore each of them in a way we may never have done before. Think of this as an adventure, an expedition into the unexplored frontiers of your own perception. I assure you that what you discover will be as surprising as it is enriching.

Let's start with sight. It is, perhaps, the sense we resort to most in our daily lives. We observe the world around us, we interpret colors, shapes, movements, and from these elements, we create our understanding of reality. However, sight can also be an obstacle to a full presence, because we are accustomed to interpret what we see through our mental and emotional filters.

To exemplify this, think of a sunset you have seen recently. Perhaps you remember the vibrant array of colors that stained the sky, the silhouettes of buildings or trees against the flaming sky. Now, imagine that you are watching that same sunset, but instead of interpreting it, you simply see it. The colors, the shapes, the shadows, everything is there, in a constant dance of light and shadow. Notice the difference?

In his book "Looking: Everyday Life Through the Eyes of a Zen Buddhist" (2010), author David Brazier highlights the importance of seeing with "fresh eyes" to experience life more fully. This ability to see without judgment, without interpretation, can have a profound impact on our tantric massage practice. Imagine being able to see your partner not as a set of expectations and judgments, but as a unique and changing being in each moment. How might this change the way you connect with him or her?

Let's turn now to the sense of hearing. Think of your favorite song, how it can evoke a wide range of emotions and memories. The ability to hear is a true blessing, and yet we often take it for granted. In our tantric massage practice, we can use listening to tune into the subtle sounds of our partner's body, heartbeat, breathing, even the tiny clicks and crackles of muscles and joints. As Alfred Tomatis pointed out in "The Ear and the Voice" (2005), our ears are a powerful tool for connection.

We continue with the sense of smell. Often underestimated, it has the ability to evoke the deepest memories and elicit strong emotional responses. Smell plays a crucial role in intimacy, as Rachel Herz points out in "The Scent of You" (2008), as it connects us on a primal, visceral level. In our tantric practice, using smell to tune into our partner's natural scent can deepen our connection and elevate our experience to new levels.

To talk about the senses without mentioning touch would be a serious omission, especially when we are talking about tantric massage. Have you ever noticed how your skin responds to the gentlest of caresses? Have you felt that electric current that runs through your body when someone you desire touches you for the first time? Touch is the language of the body, a form of communication older than words, and its power should not be underestimated. Diane Ackerman, in her "A Natural History of the Senses" (1990), explores the beauty and importance of touch in our daily lives and how it affects our perception of the world.

Last but not least, we have taste. When we eat, we experience a multitude of tastes: sweet, bitter, salty, sour, umami. But the sense of taste goes beyond the food we eat. In a tantric context, taste can be an intimate form of connection with our partner. Kissing, for example, can be a deeply sensual and connective experience, full of flavors and sensations.

Now that we have explored each of our senses, I would like to invite you to take a short pause. Close your eyes for a moment and focus your attention on your senses - what do you see, what do you hear, what do you smell, what do you touch, what do you taste? This is the basis of your presence in the moment, the gateway to full awareness and the key to a deeper and more enriching tantric practice.

Remember, this journey through your senses is not a destination, it is a journey. There is no definite end, there is only exploration and discovery. Each time you tune into your senses, you open the door to new experiences and perceptions.

This chapter has been a journey through your senses, an opportunity to rediscover the wonders that await you at the portal of the present. As always, I encourage you to explore, to experiment and to be curious. Each of your senses is a gift, a tool to help you connect with the world around you and with your partner in tantric massage.

As we move forward in our journey, we will prepare to explore the importance of the breath in the next chapter. Did you know that the breath can be a powerful tool for channeling sexual energy? And that practicing specific breathing techniques can enhance your tantric experiences? I assure you that this knowledge will be a valuable resource in your tantric journey, so don't miss the opportunity to explore this essential facet of your being.

So here we are, ready to dive deeper into this fascinating world of tantric massage. I'm excited to join you on this adventure, are you ready for the next chapter, let's go!

Chapter 4: The Breath of Life: Pranayama and Sexual Energy

Take a moment to realize something amazing. Right now, at this very moment, you are breathing. Seems obvious, doesn't it? But how many times a day do we really stop to appreciate the miracle of our breath. It is this simple, yet vital, act of inhaling and exhaling that keeps us alive, connecting us to the world around us and to ourselves. What if I told you that breath can be an incredibly powerful tool in your tantric journey? What would it feel like to know that every breath you take can be a doorway to greater intimacy, pleasure and connection?

Breathing is the key to unlocking an essential part of tantric sexual energy. In tantra, this energy is called "Prana", a Sanskrit word meaning "life force". Prana is believed to flow through everything in the universe, and to be present in each of us. This energy can be channeled and directed through the practice of Pranayama, an ancient yogic breathing technique that translates as "prana control".

The practice of Pranayama is not just a way of breathing; it is a path to greater awareness, a way to connect more deeply with your body and your sexual energy. As yoga teacher and author Donna Farhi says in her book "The Breathing Book" (1996), "Breathing is the thread that connects all aspects of our lives, from our ability to work efficiently to our ability to remember, feel, think and create."

So how can you begin to experiment with the breath in your tantric practice? Before exploring specific breathing techniques, it is important to first familiarize yourself with your own breath. Take a moment to focus on your breath. How does your breath feel right now? Is it shallow or deep? Fast or slow? Are you breathing primarily through your nose or your mouth?

Explore your breath without judging it. Just observe. By becoming aware of your breath, you are already taking an important step toward greater connection with yourself and your sexual energy. Remember, every breath you take is an act of life, a constant cycle of giving and receiving that reflects the dance of sexual energy. And here, in this chapter, I will guide you in how you can begin to dance with your breath, to play with it, to direct it and unleash its potential for deeper pleasure and connection.

So now, let's breathe together and embark on this journey of exploration and discovery of the power of the breath in tantric practice. Are you ready to discover the hidden potential in every breath you take?

You may wonder then, what is this pranayama we are talking about? The term pranayama is derived from the Sanskrit "prana", which means "vital energy" or "life force", and "ayama", which means "control" or "expansion". Thus, pranayama is literally the expansion and control of vital energy through the breath.

In his classic book "Light on Pranayama" (1981), the renowned yogi B.K.S. Iyengar describes pranayama as "the art of breath regulation". He explains that by regulating our breathing, we can regulate our mind and our emotional state. Furthermore, by mastering pranayama, we can awaken and channel our vital energy, or prana, through our bodies and our lives. Thus, pranayama is more than just a breathing technique; it is a powerful tool for personal and spiritual transformation.

The practice of pranayama involves various breathing techniques, each with its own benefits and purposes. Some techniques help to calm the mind, others to energize the body, and others still to balance our internal energies. What they all have in common is that they teach us to breathe consciously and deliberately. Do you realize how this can be crucial in our tantric exploration?

In tantra, pranayama is used to help awaken and control sexual energy, and to facilitate its movement through the chakras or energy centers of the body. And yes, we will talk more in depth about the chakras in a later chapter. But for now, understand that through pranayama, you can learn to guide this powerful energy, bringing it from the base of the spine, where it is usually dormant, to the crown chakra at the top of your head.

Writer and tantra teacher Margot Anand, in her book "The Art of Sexual Ecstasy" (1989), discusses how pranayama can be used to increase and control sexual energy, which in turn can lead to more intense and longer-lasting orgasms, and a greater sense of connection with oneself and others.

So on this journey we are embarking on together, I invite you to explore the pranayama techniques I will guide you through below. These practices can change the way you experience your body, your energy and your sexuality. Are you ready to breathe deeply and dive into the depths of your life energy? Are you ready to awaken and channel your life force through the simple yet powerful practice of conscious breathing? Let's do this together. Breathe with me.

Now, let's let the theory breathe a little and move on to practice. Let me show you a couple of pranayama techniques that you can easily integrate into your daily routine. But first, I want you to find a comfortable place where you can sit or lie down without distractions. It can be your couch, your bed, a yoga mat, or even a place outdoors if the weather permits. Once you've found your spot, take a moment to relax and focus on your body. Feel that sense of calm begin to wash over you? That's a good start. Ready for more? Here we go!

The first technique I would like to share with you is Deep Breathing Pranayama. It is a simple but incredibly effective exercise to calm the mind and increase body awareness.

To begin, place one hand on your abdomen and the other on your chest. Close your eyes and begin to inhale deeply through your nose, feeling your abdomen rise. Imagine that you are filling a water bottle from the bottom up. As you fill your inner "bottle," your chest will expand after your abdomen. Pause briefly, then exhale slowly, feeling your chest and abdomen deflate. Repeat this breathing cycle for a few minutes, allowing yourself to feel each inhale and exhale. Do you feel how this simple act of conscious breathing is already bringing you a sense of calm and connection?

The second exercise I want to share with you is the Alternate Nostril Breathing Pranayama, also known as Nadi Shodhana. This technique is especially useful for balancing the masculine and feminine energies within us, a topic we will explore further in Chapter 8.

To do Nadi Shodhana, begin by closing your eyes and taking a deep breath. Then, using the thumb of your right hand, gently close your right nostril and inhale through your left nostril. At the end of the inhalation, close the left nostril with the ring or middle finger of the same hand, release the thumb and exhale through the right nostril. Then, inhale through the right nostril, close it with the thumb, release the ring or middle finger and exhale through the left nostril. Repeat this cycle for a few minutes.

Writer and yogini Shiva Rea, in her book "Tending the Heart Fire: Living in Flow with the Pulse of Life" (2014), talks about how Nadi Shodhana can help "cleanse and purify the body's energy channels, allowing energy to flow freely." Do you feel how this practice brings you balance and serenity?

Each of these pranayama exercises can be a powerful tool in your tantric path, allowing you to take control of your vital and sexual energy. I encourage you to explore them and see for yourself. See if they provide you with a sense of deeper connection to your sexual and vital energy. Remember, there is no right or wrong way to do this. It's all about exploring and finding what works for you.

Now, you might ask, why is this connection with our breath so relevant? What does all this have to do with tantric massage? Well, the answer is quite simple and at the same time deeply complex. The breath is the vehicle through which we channel our vital energy, our sexual energy. When we learn to control and understand our breath, we begin to have a much greater mastery of our sexual energy. And it is precisely this energy that we use during tantric massage to reach states of awareness and pleasure never before experienced.

In his work "The Radiance Sutras: 112 Gateways to the Yoga of Wonder and Delight" (2014), Lorin Roche teaches us that "the breath is the constant flow of the divine in you, the living current of love that nourishes life." When we learn to breathe consciously, we become expert navigators in the current of our own life energy, allowing us to surf the waves of tantric ecstasy.

I hope this exploration of pranayama has provided you with a new set of tools to help you on your tantric path. I invite you to continue to practice these techniques and observe how they influence your daily life and your tantric massage practice. But don't worry if it seems complicated or disconcerting at first. As with any new skill, practice makes perfect. And remember, I'm always here to help you along the way.

In the next chapter, we will take a step further in our journey of self-discovery and dive into the wonderful world of self-care and nutrition. We will talk about how to honor our body as the sacred temple it is, nourishing it both physically and spiritually. I'll show you how the food you eat, the thoughts you think and the way you take care of yourself can greatly affect your sexual energy. So take a deep breath, my brave explorer of ecstasy, and get ready to delve further into the waters of tantra. Are you ready for the journey?

Chapter 5: The Body as Temple: Self-Care and Nutrition

Welcome back, brave traveler on the path of tantra. Have you been practicing the pranayama techniques we explored in the last chapter? Have you noticed a new current of energy flowing through your body, a greater sense of connection with your deeper self? It's wonderful to see you again, full of curiosity and ready to continue exploring.

Today we are going to address a crucial topic, which is often ignored in our hectic modern society. It is about self-care and nutrition, and how these relate to our vital and sexual energy. In this tantric path, our body is our temple, the sacred vehicle through which we experience and celebrate life. And like any temple, it needs to be cared for, revered and nurtured so that it can function at its fullest capacity.

Have you ever thought about how amazing your body is? Every cell, every tissue, every organ working in perfect harmony to keep us alive and functioning. The way our heart beats, our lungs breathe, our brain processes information, is a miracle of nature, an amazing testament to the wisdom and beauty of the universe.

So what are we doing to honor this incredible gift we have been given? Are we taking care of our body with the love and attention it deserves? Are we feeding it the nutrients it needs to flourish and thrive? Or are we mistreating it with processed foods, lack of sleep, stress and lack of exercise?

Remember, the path of tantra is not just about breathing techniques and erotic massage. It is about a way of life, a path of total acceptance and love for oneself. And this includes learning to take care of our body, to nurture and love it on all levels.

The wise Persian philosopher and poet Rumi put it beautifully when he said, "Your body is not outside of you, but you are inside your body." This concept is fundamental to our exploration today. Our body is not something separate from us, but we are our body. Every thought we think, every emotion we feel, every food we eat, has a direct impact on our body and, therefore, on our vital and sexual energy.

Therefore, I invite you to start looking at your body with new eyes. Observe how it feels, how it moves, how it responds to different stimuli. What kind of food makes it feel good? What kind of exercise does it like? What kind of rest does it need? What kind of care does it crave?

You may be wondering how you can start taking care of your body in a more conscious and loving way. Well, the answer is simple, but not necessarily easy. It takes time, patience and commitment. It takes a desire to change, to live in a healthier, more balanced way. And it takes a willingness to listen to your body and honor its needs.

Fortunately, you are not alone in this journey. There is a vast amount of knowledge and wisdom available to help you on this journey. There are doctors and nutritionists, fitness trainers and massage therapists, yogis and meditation teachers, all of whom have something valuable to offer. And, of course, you have the most valuable treasure of all, your own body, your own self, which is full of wisdom and knowledge.

For example, the famous physician and author Deepak Chopra, in his book "Quantum Healing" (1989), talks about our body's incredible ability to heal itself, and how we can support this process through proper nutrition, regular exercise, sufficient rest and stress reduction. Isn't it wonderful to know that we have so much power over our own health and well-being?

Have you heard of the concept of "living food"? Living foods are foods that are full of vital energy, prana. They are foods that are as close as possible to their natural state, unprocessed and unaltered. Fresh fruits and vegetables, grains and legumes, nuts and seeds, seaweed, herbs and spices are all examples of living foods.

According to tantric philosophy, by eating these foods, we are not only nourishing our physical body, but also our vital and sexual energy. Every bite we take is an opportunity to increase our prana, our vital energy.

In his book "Diet for a New America" (1987), activist and author John Robbins talks extensively about the benefits of a plant-based diet, both for our health and the environment. And best of all, these foods are not only good for us, they are also delicious.

And this is where self-care comes in. Self-care is not just about eating right and exercising, it's also about enjoying life, about honoring our needs and desires, about treating ourselves with love and kindness.

Do you like spicy food? Then enjoy a delicious curry full of spices. Do you love chocolate? Then indulge in a piece of cocoa-rich dark chocolate. Need a day off? Then give yourself permission to relax and do what makes you feel good.

This is the true meaning of self-care. It's not about following a strict diet or a grueling exercise regimen. It's about listening to your body, honoring your needs and desires, treating yourself with love and kindness.

And, of course, self-care also includes taking care of our sexual energy. Through the tantric practices we have been exploring, we can learn to take care of our sexual energy, to cultivate and nurture it. Through conscious breathing, erotic massage, meditation, we can learn to honor our sexuality, to celebrate it, to live it fully.

Let's think of a practical, tangible example to better illustrate how self-care and nutrition affect our bodies and, ultimately, our sexual energy. Imagine you have a high-end car, a sleek and powerful vehicle. You wouldn't fill it with low-quality fuel, would you? You would understand that to maintain its performance and longevity, you would need to provide it with the best fuel, perform regular maintenance and treat it with care and respect.

Now, your body is infinitely more sophisticated and valuable than any luxury car, so doesn't it deserve at least the same level of care and attention?

Let's take the concept of "living foods" we mentioned earlier. Have you ever wondered how you would feel if your diet consisted mostly of foods full of life and energy, rather than processed and artificial foods?

Dr. Gabriel Cousens, in his book "Conscious Eating" (2000), highlights the importance of a conscious diet based on raw foods. According to him, raw and organic foods not only provide the necessary nutrients for our body, but also help to maintain and improve our energy level and vitality. The reason for this is that these foods are full of prana, the vital energy that permeates the entire universe and is the basis of our existence.

Now, what does this mean for you as a tantra practitioner? It means that you can use food as a tool to increase your sexual energy. By nourishing your body with living food, you are also nourishing your life and sexual force, you are feeding your inner fire.

So why not try incorporating more living foods into your diet? Fresh fruits and vegetables, nuts and seeds, legumes and whole grains, all of these foods are full of life and energy. And most importantly, they're full of flavor. Flavor, after all, is an essential part of the human experience, and something that is celebrated in tantra.

But remember, self-care goes beyond just nutrition. It also involves taking care of your mind and spirit. It involves taking time for yourself, to relax and rejuvenate. It involves following your passions and doing the things you love. It involves surrounding yourself with supportive and encouraging people.

For example, have you ever tried yoga or meditation? Both practices can be extremely beneficial to your overall health and well-being. Yoga not only improves your flexibility and strength, but also helps you connect with your body and sexual energy in a deeper way. Meditation, on the other hand, can help you calm your mind, reduce stress and increase your awareness of yourself and the world around you.

In his book "Light on Yoga" (1966), celebrated yoga master B.K.S. Iyengar writes about how yoga can help balance and harmonize the body and mind, creating a sense of inner peace and harmony. Through yoga and meditation, we can learn to listen to our body, honor its needs and care for it in the way it deserves.

Of course, not all forms of self-care have to be so structured or formal. Something as simple as taking a relaxing bath, reading a book you enjoy, or spending time in nature can also have a profound effect on your well-being and sexual energy.

Dr. Christiane Northrup, in her book "Women's Bodies, Women's Wisdom" (1994), discusses the importance of self-care rituals in our daily lives. According to her, when we take the time to care for ourselves, we not only improve our health and well-being, but we also connect more deeply with our essence and our sexual energy.

Because at the end of the day, self-care is not a luxury, it is a necessity. It is an essential part of our health and well-being, and an integral part of our tantric practice.

We have traveled together through the lands of self-care and nutrition, discovering how our body, this sacred temple, is nourished and cared for in order to harbor the tantric energy that yearns to awaken. We have talked, we have reflected, and I hope you have learned as well. But our journey is just beginning.

Now, imagine for a moment? What if we could unlock an inexhaustible source of energy within us? What would it be like if that energy could lift us to levels of consciousness and ecstasy never before experienced? That, dear reader, is exactly what we will explore in our next chapter.

In Chapter 6, "Kundalini Awakens: Sexual Energy and Spirituality", we will delve into the mysteries of kundalini energy, a powerful and transformative life force that resides in each of us. We will learn how to awaken it and how to channel it to improve our sexual and spiritual life.

I am excited to continue this journey with you. To become fellow travelers on this path of ecstasy. So, are you ready to continue, are you ready to discover the secrets your body has been waiting to reveal to you? If so, take a deep breath, open your heart and join me on the next chapter of this extraordinary tantric adventure.

Until then, always remember: your body is a temple, and it deserves to be cared for and honored as such. Because, after all, the path to ecstasy begins with loving and caring for yourself.

Chapter 6: Kundalini Awakens: Sexual Energy and Spirituality

As we move forward in our journey, I invite you to prepare yourself to discover a new dimension, a new level of consciousness and ecstasy. But what exactly is it that awaits us? What is that hidden power within us, waiting to be awakened?

The answer, dear reader, is Kundalini, the sacred energy that lies at our base, waiting to be awakened to unleash our fullest potential, our sexual and spiritual energy. Why is this energy so important? What can it do for you, for your life, for your well-being, for your spiritual growth?

Imagine that within you is a powerful river, a torrent of latent energy that has the capacity to transform you, to elevate your consciousness, to intensify your pleasure. That river is the Kundalini, the vital and sexual energy that runs through your spine, from the base to the crown. And when it is awakened, when that river is released, you experience life, sexuality and spirituality in a completely new and revolutionary way.

According to ancient yogic traditions, Kundalini is the universal cosmic energy that lies dormant at the base of the spine, symbolized as a coiled serpent. When awakened, this energy ascends through the chakras, illuminating them and uniting our physical being with the divine.

So the question is, how can we awaken this energy? How can we unleash that inner power and connect with our deepest essence, with our inherent divinity?

Well, this is where tantric massage comes into play. Through tantric practices, we can learn to unlock and awaken the Kundalini, releasing our spiritual and sexual potential.

Remember when we talked in Chapter 4 about Pranayama, breathing and sexual energy? At that time, we barely skimmed the surface of what this powerful energy can do. Now, it's time to go deeper, to delve into the mystery and power of Kundalini.

At this stage of our journey, I invite you to keep an open mind, a willing heart and a curious spirit. It doesn't matter if some of the concepts seem a bit abstract or difficult to understand at first. Remember, we are exploring new, unknown territory. It's normal to feel a little lost or overwhelmed. But don't worry, I am here with you, guiding you step by step on this path to ecstasy.

And now, are you ready to awaken your Kundalini, to release your sexual and spiritual energy? Are you ready to transform your life and your being in a way you never imagined possible? If so, let's take a deep breath, relax and step into the mystery of Kundalini.

The concept of Kundalini and its awakening features prominently in the literature of many spiritual traditions around the world, but it is the Vedic texts of ancient India that give us the most complete and detailed insight into this phenomenon. In these texts, Kundalini is often described as a powerful sleeping serpent coiled at the base of the spine. Don't you find it fascinating, this ancient metaphor that speaks to us of such an immense power dormant within us, waiting for the moment of its awakening?

You are probably asking yourself, what does all this have to do with spirituality and sexuality? Philosopher and psychologist Carl Jung, in his work "The Psychological Aspects of Kundalini Yoga" (1932), provides a useful framework for understanding this connection. According to Jung, Kundalini is not only a source of vital energy, but also a symbolic representation of the psychological and spiritual development of the individual. Don't you think this is an extraordinary insight?

Kundalini awakening, then, can not only provide renewed sexual vigor and a greater sense of vitality, but it can also open us to a new dimension of spiritual experience. As it moves up the spine and activates each of the chakras, Kundalini energy can provide a sense of oneness with the universe, a feeling of being in harmony with the flow of life. Can you imagine what it would be like to feel something like that?

However, this process is not always easy. Awakening Kundalini can be a challenging journey, full of ups and downs. As Gopi Krishna, a famous yogi and mystic who described his own Kundalini awakening experience in "Kundalini: The Evolutionary Energy in Man" (1967), warns us, the path can be difficult and requires careful preparation and proper guidance.

But tantric massage, with its emphasis on conscious connection, breath and touch, can be a very effective tool for facilitating this process. Through tantric massage, you can learn to channel your sexual energy, release blockages and awaken and direct Kundalini energy. Don't you think it's wonderful to have such a powerful tool for personal and spiritual growth at your disposal?

Allow me to accompany you a little more on this journey, and together we will explore the techniques and practices that can help you awaken your Kundalini. Remember, this is not a race, but a journey of discovery and transformation. So, are you ready to continue?

Good! I'm excited that you're here, ready to delve even deeper into this intriguing path. Can you imagine the Kundalini energy like a snake uncoiling, surging powerfully from deep within you, activating each of your energy centers in its wake, until it finally reaches the top of your head, and suddenly, everything becomes clear, consciousness expands and oneness with the universe becomes present? It's a striking idea, don't you think?

Now, we must understand that the awakening of Kundalini is a process that requires attention and care. It is not something we should force or rush. This is where tantric massage comes into play. Through the practices and techniques of tantric massage, it is possible to learn to channel sexual energy, release blockages and cultivate a state of presence that can facilitate the awakening of Kundalini.

Let's look at a practical example. Imagine you are in a tantric massage session. You are lying in a calm and welcoming environment, your body and mind are completely relaxed, and the person massaging you is applying gentle pressure at various points along your spine, following the path of the Kundalini energy. With each touch, you can feel the tension release, the energy begin to move and flow more freely. It is as if your body is getting rid of old blockages and restrictions, preparing for the awakening of the Kundalini.

Can you visualize it, can you feel that sense of release and flow? This is the power of tantric massage. And while this is just one example, actual practice can vary considerably depending on individual needs and the guidance of a trained practitioner.

Lizelle Le Roux, in her book "Kundalini Tantra Yoga: Journey within through the Chakras" (2019), offers an in-depth look at practices that can help awaken Kundalini. According to Le Roux, a safe and effective Kundalini awakening requires holistic preparation that encompasses both mind and body.

So how can you prepare for this awakening? Well, one way is through the regular practice of tantric massage, as I mentioned earlier. But there are other tools that can complement and enhance this process, such as meditation, conscious breathing, healthy eating, physical exercise and exploring your own emotional blocks and thought patterns.

Don't worry if this all seems a little overwhelming now. The important thing is that you're on the right path. You are here, willing to learn and grow, and that is a wonderful thing. Let's move forward, and together we will explore even more of this fascinating journey towards Kundalini awakening. Are you ready?

Without a doubt, this journey we are sharing is incredibly fascinating. As you may have noticed, the awakening of Kundalini is not just a matter of energy and physiology. It is a delicate and sublime dance, an interaction between mind, body and spirit. It is not simply a matter of awakening a latent energy within you, but of embracing a new level of awareness and connection with everything around you.

Tantric massage, as we have discovered, is a powerful tool in this process. Through its techniques and its focus on presence and connection, it allows us to release blockages and resistances, encourage the flow of energy and open us to the possibility of experiencing the ecstasy of Kundalini awakening.

Let me give you one more example to solidify this idea. Suppose you are in the middle of a dance, moving to the beat of the music. But you are not alone. Your dance partner is your own Kundalini energy, and every step, every turn, every movement is an expression of that energy. Sometimes the dance is calm and gentle. Other times, it is passionate and frenetic. But always, always, it is a dance of union, of integration, of being one with the music, one with the energy, one with all that exists.

A notable reference is Gopi Krishna's "Kundalini: The Evolutionary Energy in Man" (1967), in which he recounts his own experience with Kundalini awakening and provides valuable insight into this phenomenon. Krishna reminds us that the awakening of Kundalini, although it can be challenging and at times disconcerting, is ultimately a gift, an opportunity to expand our consciousness and experience life in a deeper and more meaningful way.

So here we are, at the end of this chapter, ready to continue our journey. Can you feel the excitement, the anticipation? But also, can you feel the calm, the peace that comes with knowing you are on the right path? I hope so, because in the next chapter, we will delve into a very important aspect of this journey: the art of surrender. We will learn how to overcome blocks and resistances and how to fully open ourselves to the experience of tantric massage and Kundalini awakening.

I'm excited to share this with you. Because remember, you are not alone on this journey. I'm here with you, one step at a time, one breath at a time. And together, we're going to discover, we're going to learn, we're going to grow. Are you ready for the next step? I assure you, it will be a journey you will never forget.

Chapter 7: The Art of Surrender: Overcoming Blockages and Resistance

The path to ecstasy and tantric enlightenment is one that winds through mountains and valleys, through dark forests and sun-drenched meadows. But what happens when you encounter an obstacle in your path, a high and imposing wall that seems impassable? Do you give up? Do you turn around and look for another way? Or do you find the strength and courage to overcome this blockage and continue your journey?

This is an important question that we all face at some point in our lives. And in the context of tantric massage and Kundalini awakening, it is a question that takes on an even deeper meaning. In this chapter, we will explore the art of surrender, the ability to overcome blockages and resistances, physical, emotional and spiritual. You will see why this is an essential skill for any seeker of tantra and how you can cultivate it in your own life.

Why is delivery so important, and why can it be so difficult to achieve?

Surrender is important because it allows us to release tensions, fears and worries that can hinder the flow of Kundalini energy. It is the key that opens the door to deeper intimacy, truer connection, and fuller awakening. But at the same time, surrender can be challenging because it often asks us to face and release ingrained patterns and beliefs, to let go of our control and trust the process.

As the famous psychologist Carl Jung mentioned in "The Archetypes and the Collective Unconscious" (1959), "What you deny subdues you. What you accept transforms you. This quote perfectly reflects the power of surrender. By facing and accepting our resistances, we have the opportunity to transform them and release the energy held in them.

On the other hand, have you ever wondered why we have resistances and blockages in the first place? Resistance can arise for a variety of reasons, from physical or emotional trauma to cultural and social conditioning. For example, many of us have learned to repress our sexuality, to see it as shameful or impure. This belief can cause a blockage in the second chakra, the sacral chakra, which is the center of our sexuality and creativity.

Remember how in Chapter 5 we talked about self-care and nurturing? That self-care and awareness can help heal and release these resistances, allowing for a freer and healthier flow of energy.

The good news is that, despite these challenges, delivery is a skill that can be learned and cultivated. Like a muscle, surrender gets stronger with practice. And as you become more comfortable and confident in surrender, you will find that it becomes easier to overcome blocks and resistance and open to the fullness of the tantric experience.

Learning to let go, to surrender and accept, is not just a skill, it is an art. Have you ever watched the way a river flows through a landscape? It doesn't try to climb the mountains or traverse the rocks, it simply goes around them, it follows its path. This is the essence of surrender: following the course of life with confidence, even when the path may seem difficult or uncertain.

In the realm of tantric massage, surrender means allowing yourself to feel and fully experience every touch, every sensation. It means opening up to your partner and yourself, trusting the process and allowing the energy to flow freely.

Writer and spirituality teacher Marianne Williamson put it beautifully in her book "A Return to Love" (1992): "When we surrender to God, we surrender to something greater than ourselves, to a force of love that is greater than our personalities. When we surrender to God, we become more of who we are." And, we might add, more than we thought we could be.

So how can we practice the art of surrender? How can we learn to release our blocks and resistances?

One of the keys to surrender is awareness. It is about being present in each moment, observing our reactions and emotions without judgment. Remember in Chapter 3 when we talked about rediscovering our five senses? This mindful approach can be equally applied here. By paying attention to our resistances, we can begin to understand them, to understand what is blocking us.

It is important to remember that surrender does not mean being passive or letting go of our limits. Quite the opposite. It means having the courage to face our fears and blocks, and the strength to release them. As the poet and philosopher Rumi said so well in his work "The Essential Rumi" (1273): "The moment you accept what troubles you, freedom begins".

Another effective strategy for surrender is the practice of meditation and mindful breathing. By focusing our attention on the breath, we can help calm the mind, release tension and open ourselves to the experience of the present moment.

In short, surrender is a process that involves acceptance, courage and awareness. By practicing these skills, we can learn to overcome our blocks and resistances, allowing energy to flow freely and experience life in its fullness. So, are you ready to embark on this exciting journey of self-discovery and transformation?

We have talked about how surrender is fundamental in tantric massage and how you can start practicing it. Now, it is time to look in detail at how you can overcome your blocks and resistances.

Imagine for a moment that you are standing in front of an enormous, impenetrable wall. That wall represents your fears, your insecurities, the resistances that have prevented you from giving yourself fully in your life. How do you feel when you see that wall? Threatened? Embarrassed? Frustrated? Remember, it's normal to feel all this. But now, I want you to do something different. Instead of trying to break down that wall, what you will do is open a door.

As Carl Jung, famous Swiss psychologist and psychiatrist, expressed in "Man and His Symbols" (1964), "What you deny subdues you, what you accept transforms you". So by opening the door to your own resistance, instead of trying to fight it, you can begin to work with it and transform it.

And how can you do this? One way is by consciously exploring your resistances. When you find yourself struggling with certain sensations or emotions during a tantric massage session, pause and breathe. Try to observe what is going on inside you without judging yourself. Is there a specific fear that is surfacing? An old memory that is causing pain? A limiting belief that is impeding your progress?

Another way is through open and honest communication with your partner. Express your fears and concerns. Talk about your limits and your expectations. Your partner cannot read your mind, and the only way to overcome your resistance is to face it together.

And finally, remember to practice patience and kindness with yourself. Overcoming blocks and resistance is not an overnight process. It takes time, effort and, most importantly, a compassionate attitude toward yourself. As Thich Nhat Hanh, the renowned Zen master, said in "Being Peace" (1987), "Compassion for oneself is the basis for compassion for others." Therefore, be kind to yourself. You are a human being, and it is okay to be afraid and feel resistance. What matters is that you are here, you are trying, and you are willing to grow.

So, are you ready to open that door and start transforming your resistances into growth and self-knowledge? Remember, the journey may be difficult, but I promise you it will be worth it. After all, as the tantric proverb says: "The lotus blooms in the mud". And you, dear reader, are on the path to bloom in your inner lotus.

And so, you have reached the end of this profound and important chapter. In this journey through the art of surrender, you have explored the concepts of blockages and resistances, faced your fears and opened the door to overcome them. Through this work of self-knowledge and self-exploration, you are becoming the master of your own being, capable of handling whatever difficulties life throws at you.

Let me remind you that surrender is an art, an act of courage. It requires trust in oneself and in the other. It is a constant journey of introspection, self-acceptance and self-care. True surrender is not renunciation, it is full participation, it is being fully present in every moment, every sensation, every emotion. As the poet and philosopher Ralph Waldo Emerson said in "Self-Reliance" (1841): "Trust yourself: every heart vibrates with that iron cord".

There may be days when you feel overwhelmed by your blocks and resistances, but I want you to remember one thing: every step you take, no matter how small, is a step towards liberation. Don't give up. Don't get discouraged. You are on the right path. And I promise you, once you have overcome your resistances and surrender to the wonder of tantric massage, you will experience a sense of freedom and empowerment like never before.

I am excited for you, dear reader. I am excited for the discoveries you are about to make, for the transformations you are about to experience. And you know what? This is just the beginning.

In the next chapter, we will explore the intriguing play of polarity and the fascinating dance between the masculine and feminine. You'll discover how these two aspects, often thought of as opposites, can come together to create a magnificent and magical synergy. Ready to discover how polarity can intensify your tantric experience and elevate it to new levels of ecstasy and understanding? I assure you, you won't want to miss what's to come.

So, take my hand, let's take one more step in this fascinating journey into the heart of tantric massage. With every word you read, you are opening your world to new possibilities, you are getting closer and closer to your true self. Don't look back now, the best is yet to come, see you in the next chapter!

Chapter 8: The Polarity Game: Exploring Masculine and Feminine

Since the dawn of humanity, the duality of the masculine and feminine has been a fundamental part of our existence, forming the foundation of our understanding of the world. But have you ever stopped to really consider what these forces represent and how they interact with each other? What if I told you that this understanding could be the key to opening the door to a richer and deeper tantric experience?

We are constantly surrounded by the forces of the masculine and the feminine, both in the external world and within ourselves. These are not merely references to the biological sexes, but are energies, principles, that are found in all things, in all people, regardless of gender. And each of us carries a unique blend of these energies within us. Have you ever wondered how these forces balance within you? What would happen if you set out to explore them, embrace them, integrate them?

Taoism, an ancient philosophy and spiritual system of China, described these two forces as Yin and Yang, illustrated in the familiar circle divided into black and white. According to the Chinese philosopher Lao Tzu in the "Tao Te Ching" (6th century B.C.), "Everything has Yin and possesses Yang." Yin, associated with the feminine, represents the dark, the receptive, the intuitive. Yang, associated with the masculine, represents the light, the active, the logical.

Yoga also recognizes this duality through the idea of Shiva and Shakti. According to the ancient Vedic texts of the "Rig

Veda" (1700-1100 B.C.), Shiva represents pure consciousness, the masculine principle, while Shakti represents creative energy and life force, the feminine principle. Together, they give form to all reality.

How do these forces manifest in you? At what times do you feel you are more in your masculine, logical energy, and at what times do you feel more in your feminine, intuitive energy? There is no right or wrong answer to these questions. And through exploring these energies in yourself and in your partner, you can begin to better understand your own nature and enjoy a deeper, more rewarding relationship.

In tantric massage, we play with this duality, creating a dance between the masculine and feminine, allowing these energies to flow and intertwine in a way that magnifies the experience for both. In this dance, you can explore the roles of giving and receiving, leading and following, and discover how these interactions affect your experience of pleasure and connection.

This exploration can bring about a deeper understanding of oneself and one's partner, and can open up new possibilities for pleasure and connection. And, as we explore this play of polarity, we can also begin to discover how this dance extends beyond our bodies and manifests in all aspects of our lives.

You may be asking yourself, how do I begin to explore this polarity within myself and in my interactions with others? Well, the answer is through awareness. Yes, the same awareness that we have been cultivating throughout this tantric journey. And, remember when we talked in Chapter 3 about the importance of rediscovering your five senses as a portal to the present? Now we can take that awareness a step further and apply it to our understanding of the masculine and feminine polarity in our lives.

The psychologist Carl Jung, in his work "Aion: Researches into the Phenomenology of the Self" (1951), spoke of the importance of recognizing and integrating the masculine and feminine aspects of our psyche, which he called the anima and animus. He argued that each individual carries within him or herself these two forces and that our task is to bring them into the light of consciousness and allow them to express themselves, balancing each other.

So what does this look like in practice? It could be as simple as paying attention to how you behave in different situations. Are there times when you feel more active, more purposeful, more focused on logic and action, thus manifesting the masculine or Yang energy in you? And what about when you feel more receptive, more intuitive, more focused on emotions and sensations, manifesting the feminine or Yin energy in you? How does each of these states feel? How do they affect your interactions with others? And how does your experience change when you allow yourself to shift from one energy to the other?

Remembering Jung's words, there is nothing wrong with expressing one energy more than the other. It is not about seeking perfection or perfect balance, but about recognizing and honoring the different parts of yourself.

While we are exploring Yin and Yang, masculine and feminine, don't be fooled by social stereotypes or preconceived notions. This is not a role-play in which the man must always be Yang and the woman always Yin. In fact, Tantra invites us to explore and celebrate all facets of our identity and to recognize that each of us contains both the light of day and the darkness of night.

And when you can embrace these opposing energies within yourself, you give yourself the freedom to play, to explore, to discover new aspects of yourself and your capacity for pleasure and connection. And that is a truly beautiful thing.

So I encourage you to give yourself the opportunity to explore this game of polarity. As the Persian poet Rumi would say in his work "Masnavi" (1268-1273), "The task is not in seeking love, but in seeking and finding all the barriers within oneself that one has built against it." So, if you please, let's continue our journey towards self-discovery and the expansion of self-love and understanding.

Now, let me paint you an image, one that will help illustrate how these polarity energies can be experienced and explored in the practice of tantric massage.

Imagine a dance. A dance of two, moving together in a dance of polarities. In this scenario, one of the participants adopts an active posture, a posture of giving, of leading. This is the Yang energy at play, the masculine principle we spoke of earlier. The other, on the other hand, adopts a receptive posture, a posture of receiving, of following. Here we see Yin energy, the feminine principle. This dance is tantric massage, a game of giving and receiving, of leading and following, of exploring the polarity between Yin and Yang energies.

But make no mistake, we are not necessarily talking about a man and a woman in this dance. As we mentioned before, these energies are independent of gender. A man can embrace his Yin energy and a woman her Yang energy. The beauty lies in the exchange and balance, in the flow of these energies between the two participants.

The famous psychologist Erich Fromm, in his book "The Art of Loving" (1956), stated that "love is an act of faith, and whoever has little faith also has little love". In this context, the giving and receiving in tantric massage is an act of love and trust, a journey towards exploration and understanding of oneself and the other.

Now, you may ask, how does one experience this dance of polarities in tantric massage? Well, it is as simple and yet as profound as presence. To be truly present, with all your awareness, in every touch, in every sigh, in every glance. To feel how the energy flows from you to the other and vice versa, to feel how the polarity moves and changes, and to allow yourself to flow with it.

Of course, this dance of polarities is not limited to tantric massage. It extends to all areas of our lives. When we are able to understand, to integrate, to embrace our masculine and feminine energies, we become more complete, more balanced. We become able to relate to ourselves and others in a more authentic and empathic way.

And now, my dear reader, are you willing to dance this dance of polarities? Are you willing to explore and embrace all parts of yourself? I promise you it is a journey worth taking.

And so, we look up and see how the dance of polarities has led us to a new horizon. But, dear friend, we have not reached our destination. On the contrary, each step we take opens a new and exciting path on this journey that is tantra.

We have walked the paths of polarity and delighted in its dance. We have explored the intrinsic nature of our masculine and feminine energies, and how they can flow and balance each other in the practice of tantric massage.

The philosopher Alan Watts, in his work "The Wisdom of Insecurity" (1951), proclaimed that "the only way to make sense of a change is to immerse yourself in it, move with it, and join the dance". Thus, by allowing ourselves to flow with the energies, by joining the dance, we are accessing a greater understanding of ourselves and our relationship with the universe.

And, in this context, tantric massage is presented as an invitation to this wonderful dance of energies, where each movement is another step towards the connection with our most authentic self and with the other.

But, dear reader, our journey is far from over. In the next chapter, we will dive even deeper into tantric energy as we explore how tantra can be practiced as a couple. And, yes, you can expect this part of the journey to be filled with more magic, more discoveries and, of course, more love.

For now, I encourage you to reflect on what we have explored in this chapter. How can you incorporate these concepts of polarity into your daily life? How can you open yourself to the dance of energies within yourself and with others? These are questions that, I hope, will invite you to think, grow, and move forward on this journey toward tantric wholeness.

And now, with my heart full of gratitude for your company on this journey, I invite you to take a step forward. Are you ready, dear friend, to continue dancing together in this wonderful dance of tantra? Because remember, in this journey there are no limits, only horizons waiting to be discovered. Until the next chapter, my friend.

Chapter 9: Dancing with the Energy: The Practice of Tantra in Couples

We enter this new chapter, dear reader, as two traveling companions embarking on an exciting and transformative expedition. Together, we have explored paths of self-discovery and danced with the polarities of our essential nature. Now, we prepare to enter an even deeper territory, that of the practice of tantra as a couple.

First of all, let me ask you: Why do you think the practice of tantra as a couple is important? What does it mean to you to share this dance of energies with another person?

Well, partner tantra is important because it allows us to explore our ability to connect deeply with another human being, both on a physical and spiritual level. This practice challenges us to expand our perception of love, pleasure and intimacy, and to experience the shared ecstasy that can arise when two energies intertwine in a tantric dance.

Having said that, let's get into the essence of couple tantric practice. Remember when we talked in chapter 7 about surrender? Well, in partner tantra, this surrender takes on an additional dimension. Not only are you surrendering to the tantric energy and your own inner exploration, but you are also surrendering to the journey together with your partner.

Now, this joint surrender does not mean losing oneself in the other. Rather, it is about opening up to a shared energy field in which each of you can resonate and flow freely. In this dance, each of you is both leader and follower, each of you is both the dancer and the dance itself.

Certainly, there is something profoundly beautiful and powerful about sharing tantric dance with a partner. However, it can also be challenging, as it requires honesty, vulnerability and the ability to be present and open to each other's experience.

So I invite you to approach this practice with an attitude of curiosity and openness, willing to explore new dimensions of yourself and your relationship. And, of course, always with a sense of humor and a smile on your face. After all, tantra is a journey into joy and enjoyment, a celebration of life in all its forms.

Get ready, then, to enter into the mystery and wonder of the practice of tantra as a couple. In this chapter, we will explore together how this practice can enrich your life and relationships, weave a deeper bond of connection and open you to levels of pleasure and ecstasy you may never have imagined possible.

Are you ready, dear friend, to take this exciting step on our tantric journey? Then dive with me into the depths of tantra as a couple, and discover the transformative power of dancing with energy... together.

As we explore the practice of tantra as a couple, we discover a way of connecting that transcends the familiarity of everyday interactions. This is not simply about learning a series of techniques or postures; it is a path of discovery, an invitation to immerse ourselves in the current of shared consciousness and energy.

As Daniel Odier mentioned in his work "Desire: Tantra and Sexual Energy" (2001), "Tantra is the path of acceptance and love. It helps us to accept our own body, our emotions, our perceptions... and finally, it leads us to a state of love and acceptance towards the other. True tantra is a path of deep communion with oneself and with others." So, beloved reader, in our exploration of tantra as a couple, we are embarking on a journey towards greater authenticity, connection and love.

Let's talk now about the dynamic between giving and receiving in partnered tantra. This dance is often a balancing act, a matter of learning to navigate between the desire to give pleasure and the ability to receive it. This is where the true alchemy of tantra lies.

Recalling the teachings of Margot Anand in her book "The Art of Sexual Ecstasy: The Way of Tantra" (1989), who is known for her contributions to the modern practice of tantra, she stated: "In giving, we receive; in receiving, we give. This mutual dance of energies is what creates the circle of ecstasy." Reflect for a moment on these words, dear friend, how do they make you feel? What images or sensations do they evoke in you?

Exploring this balance can be challenging, but it can also be a path of profound growth and learning. When we open ourselves to receive, we allow our partner to express themselves through their giving. And when we give generously, we invite our partner to experience the pleasure of receiving. This mutual dance of giving and receiving can generate a circuit of energy, creating a flow that intensifies and expands as we surrender to it.

Now, dear reader, imagine this: you are in a quiet, safe space with your partner. The light is soft, the music is soft, and you are both present and aware, breathing together, synchronizing your hearts. With each breath, you feel the energy flowing between you, each reflecting and responding to the other, in a dance of give and take.

This is just a glimpse of what it can be like to practice tantra as a couple, a dance of energy and ecstasy that can take you to depths of connection and intimacy that you may never have experienced before. In the next section, we'll delve more deeply into this practice and I'll provide you with some concrete tools and techniques for exploring this dance with your partner. Are you ready to move forward? Well then, my friend, let's continue our journey.

At the heart of this dance of giving and receiving is the act of presence, of truly being there, in the moment, with your partner. No matter what technique or posture you are practicing, if you are not present, the true potential of tantra cannot flourish. Presence, as renowned tantra and yoga author Christopher Wallis mentioned in "Tantra Illuminated" (2007), "is the key to unlocking the flow of energy and consciousness."

Think about this for a moment, my friend. When you are present, truly present, everything is intensified. The colors are brighter, the sounds sharper, the flavors richer. And in contact with your partner, when you are fully there, every touch, every whisper, every glance is magnified.

Let's explore this further with a concrete example. Imagine you are caressing your partner's hand. If you are distracted, thinking about work or what you are going to do next, your stroking may be automatic, lacking true connection. But if you are fully present, if all your attention is focused on the act of caressing, every movement of your hand becomes a gesture of love, a wordless communication that says, "I'm here, with you, in this moment." Can you feel the difference? Can you imagine how powerful this can be when applied to the practice of tantra as a couple?

But how is this presence cultivated? As teacher and author Diana Richardson mentions in "The Heart of Tantric Sex" (2003), "Presence in the act of loving is cultivated through mindfulness, awareness and conscious breathing." It is a path back to yourself, a path back to the present moment. And every time you come back, you realize that everything you need is here and now.

Practicing presence can be as simple as focusing on the breath. When you realize that you have become distracted, gently, lovingly, return to your breath. This is the anchor that keeps you in the present, that keeps you grounded and connected.

With practice, you will begin to notice a change. The mind becomes calmer, the heart more open. And in this openness, you can find a space for tantric energy to flow, a space for intimacy and connection to flourish.

Dear reader, as you explore the path of tantra as a couple, remember that each step is part of the journey. There is no final destination to arrive at, only this moment, over and over again. So breathe, be present, and enjoy the dance.

In the next section, we will dive even deeper into this dance. We'll explore how you can use the techniques and practices of tantra to cultivate a stronger and more coherent flow of energy with your partner. But for now, just take a moment to reflect on what you've learned so far. How can you apply these ideas to your own partner practice? What changes can you begin to notice as you become more present in your interactions?

Continuing our exploration, let me quote another great tantric master, Daniel Odier, who in his book "Tantric Quest: An Encounter with Absolute Love" (1997), puts forward the idea that at the heart of tantra is the desire to merge with the other, to become one. In tantric couple practices, this desire for union becomes a gateway to greater awareness and energy.

The techniques and practices of tantra as a couple go beyond the simple physical act of giving and receiving pleasure. It is a journey inward, a journey to the very essence of who we are. Every touch, every sigh, every glance becomes a vehicle for this journey.

And herein lies the true beauty of tantra. In this dance of energies, in this dance of giving and receiving, we begin to discover that there is no real separation between us and our lovers. We realize that we are a reflection of each other, a mirror reflecting our own light and darkness, our own love and fear.

So, beloved reader, as you move forward on this path of tantra as a couple, I invite you to keep this idea in your heart. Remember that every encounter is an opportunity for authentic connection and growth, an opportunity to dance with the energy of life itself.

And with this, we have come to the end of our journey through Chapter 9. We have explored the meaning of the practice of tantra as a couple and how this dance of energies can lead to greater connection and awareness. But this is only the beginning, my friend. There is so much more to discover and explore on the path of tantra.

Are you ready to move on? In the next chapter, we will explore the world of the chakras, those fascinating energy centers that play a crucial role in the flow of tantric energy. You'll learn how to work with these energy centers to increase your pleasure and deepen your connection with your partner.

I'll be waiting for you in the next chapter, where we will continue together this wonderful journey to the heart of tantric massage. Come on, my friend, the adventure awaits us!

Chapter 10: The Seven Chakras: Centers of Energy and Pleasure

Imagine for a moment that you are standing in front of a majestic pipe organ, a marvel of acoustic engineering. The instrument itself is impressive, but without the energy that flows through its pipes, without the air that flows through its innumerable passages, it is simply an inert object. What if I told you that our body is similar to that pipe organ? Yes, you read that right. We are like a musical instrument and the music we play is that of our vital energy.

Now, where does this vital energy, our prana, circulate in our body? The answer to this question leads us to the fascinating subject of the chakras.

The chakras are energy centers in our body. Originating from the ancient yogic and tantric philosophy of India, these energy vortexes, seven in all, are aligned along our central axis, from the base of the spine to the crown of the head. And today, in this tenth chapter, we will dive into the world of the chakras and discover how they are intrinsically connected to our pleasure and personal growth.

But before we get into that journey, I invite you to reflect for a moment. Have you ever experienced a sense of blockage in your life, a feeling that something is not flowing as it should? Have you sometimes felt as if there is a barrier that prevents you from feeling pleasure or even, in some cases, any kind of emotion? If your answer is yes, then you may be experiencing a blockage in your chakras.

The chakras, in their optimal state, should be open and in balance, allowing energy to flow freely through them. When the chakras are blocked or imbalanced, it can lead to a range of problems, from physical to emotional. This is why the study and understanding of the chakras is so vital.

So, how about together we discover more about these energy centers and how you can work with them to unlock your potential for pleasure and self-fulfillment? Are you ready for this energetic journey, my friend?

Let's start at the beginning. Where does the term "chakra" come from? In Sanskrit, "chakra" means "wheel" or "disk". This word is used to describe these energy centers in our body because they are considered to have a circular shape and rotate with the vital energy flowing through them.

Each chakra is associated with a specific set of physical, emotional and spiritual aspects. By working with our chakras, we can address and heal these specific areas of our lives, leading to greater health, wellness and, yes, pleasure.

Now, I will ask you a question: How would you feel if you could understand, balance and empower each of these wonderful energy centers in you? Would you like to learn to play the melody of your own being, to conduct the symphony of your vital energy?

Well, you don't have to wait any longer. Let me be your guide on this musical and vibrational journey through the seven chakras.

We will start with the first chakra, known as Muladhara or root chakra. Located at the base of the spine, it is the foundation of your energy system. Its function is to provide you with a sense of security and stability. Remember Anodea Judith's book "Eastern Body, Western Mind" published in 1996? There, Judith brilliantly explained how a balanced root chakra allows you to feel grounded and secure in your body and in your life, while an imbalanced root chakra can lead you to feel disconnected and full of fears.

We continue ascending to the second chakra, Svadhisthana or sacral chakra. Located just below the navel, it is the center of creativity and sensual pleasure. It is here that our ability to feel pleasure and experience the joy of life resides. In the classic "Wheels of Life" (1987), the same author, Anodea Judith, teaches us that when this chakra is in balance, we are able to fully enjoy life and express our creativity freely.

Next, we ascend to the third chakra, Manipura or solar plexus chakra. Located in the stomach area, it is the center of your personal power and self-esteem. Remember Caroline Myss' wonderful work in "Anatomy of the Spirit" (1996)? Myss described how a balanced solar plexus chakra allows you to feel empowered and capable, while an unbalanced chakra can leave you feeling powerless and insecure.

The journey continues to the fourth chakra, Anahata or heart chakra. Located in the center of the chest, it is the center of compassion and unconditional love. According to the teaching of Paramahansa Yogananda in his monumental work "Autobiography of a Yogi" (1946), an open and balanced heart allows you to feel love and compassion towards yourself and others, while a blocked heart chakra can lead you to feel disconnected and isolated.

Wait a second, don't you think it's amazing the wisdom we've already uncovered together? And we still have three more chakras left to explore. But before we continue, I invite you to take a deep breath, to feel each of the chakras we have reviewed so far. Do you feel how the music of your vital energy begins to play a more harmonious melody? Do you feel how each note of your inner symphony vibrates with more clarity and strength?

Come on, my friend! Let's move forward in this fascinating journey into our inner self.

The fifth chakra, Vishuddha or throat chakra, is located, as its name suggests, in the throat. It is the center of communication and expression of truth. When it is in balance, you feel able to express yourself freely and authentically, without fear of being judged or rejected. Remember "The Book of Chakras" by Ambika Wauters, published in 2002? Wauters explains how a blocked throat chakra can lead to repression of personal truth and a struggle to express yourself.

The journey continues upward to the sixth chakra, Ajna or third eye chakra, which is located in the middle of the forehead, just above the space between the eyebrows. It is the center of intuition and perception beyond the physical. Have you read "The Psychic Pathway" (1991) by Sonia Choquette? There Choquette teaches us how an open third eye allows you to perceive beyond the physical, connect with your intuition and have a clearer vision of your life.

Finally, we come to the seventh chakra, Sahasrara or crown chakra, which is located at the top of the head. It is the center of spirituality and the connection to the divine. According to what Muktananda taught us in "Play of Consciousness" (1974), a balanced crown chakra allows you to feel connected to the whole, experience higher states of consciousness and live with a deep sense of purpose and meaning.

Now that we have gone through these seven energy centers together, I would like to invite you to a little experiment. Close your eyes for a moment. Imagine that each of your chakras is a flower. The root chakra flower is red and is located at the base of your spine. The sacral chakra flower is orange and is just below your navel. The solar plexus chakra flower is yellow in color and is located in your stomach area. The heart chakra flower is green in color and is in the center of your chest. The throat chakra flower is blue in color and is located in your throat. The flower of the third eye chakra is indigo in color and is in the middle of your forehead. The crown chakra flower is violet in color and is at the top of your head.

Imagine now a bright, warm light, like sunlight, bathing each of these flowers. See how, under the warmth of this light, each flower begins to open, to unfold its petals, to vibrate with more strength and clarity. Feel how this light travels throughout your body, how it penetrates each of your chakras, how it activates and balances your vital energy. Feel how, with each breath, you become more and more attuned to the music of your being.

Do you feel that harmony, do you feel that love for yourself, that connection with your most authentic self? That connection is no coincidence. It is the music of existence itself, the rhythm of the universe flowing through you. It is the energy of life dancing in each of your chakras, illuminating them, balancing them, bringing them into harmony.

Feel how each of your chakras aligns, how they connect with each other like a series of points of light running the length of your body. Each has its color, its vibration, its purpose. But together, they work in perfect harmony to attune you to the dance of the universe.

Do you feel that burst of love and gratitude overflowing from the core of your being? That is the beauty of harmony. That is the gift of living in sync with your own rhythm, your own music.

This journey through your chakras is not the end, my friend, it is only the beginning. As you learn to tune each of your chakras, to listen to their music, to dance with their energy, you become a master of your own being. You begin to live in a new dimension of harmony and ecstasy.

Each chakra, each energy center, is a doorway to a universe of pleasure and fulfillment. And the wonderful thing about these doors is that they are open to you at all times. All you need is the courage to cross them, the desire to explore, and the willingness to embrace the dance of energy flowing through you.

And there you are, with your eyes closed, listening to the music of your chakras, feeling how each one is illuminated by the light of life, how each one opens like a flower under the warmth of the sun. It is you in your highest expression, you in your fullness, you in your authentic self.

Do you feel the power of this experience? Do you feel every fiber of your being vibrating with the energy of life? That is what it means to be alive, my friend. That is what it means to dance with the energy.

In the next chapter, we will delve into the relationship between meditation and tantric massage, and how together they can help you cultivate mindfulness. How might your life change if you could be present in each moment, if you could live each experience with full awareness? Imagine the benefits you could gain from such an approach in your life. Imagine how it could improve your relationships, your work, your health, your sense of purpose.

I invite you to follow me on this exciting journey, to explore with me the wonderful universe of tantra. Because, at the end of the day, this book is not just about me sharing my knowledge with you. It's about us, exploring together, learning together, growing together. I'll be waiting for you in the next chapter, are you ready to continue this journey?

Chapter 11: Meditation and Tantric Massage: Cultivating Mindfulness

Have you ever stopped to observe how a drop of water slowly descends through a window pane on a rainy day? Have you ever realized the wonder of contemplating each instant in its complete and total individuality, of recognizing the beauty and uniqueness in each millisecond that makes up the journey of the drop of water? Isn't it wonderful and captivating?

This is the power of mindfulness, or mindfulness, as it is known in the world of psychology and mind disciplines. Mindfulness is the ability to be fully present in the moment, free from distractions and completely immersed in the experience we are living.

Why is this important? I'll explain. We live in a world that constantly pulls us into the future or makes us relive the past. Our mind is perpetually jumping from one thought to another, from one worry to another, from one memory to a plan. But how often do we really stop to live in the present? How often have you really allowed yourself to be in the here and now, free of distractions and fully present in what you are doing?

This is where mindfulness intersects with tantric massage. Like the drop of water on the windowpane, each caress in a tantric massage is an invitation to be present, to immerse ourselves in the moment and to experience the fullness of the sensory experience.

But before we dive into the depths of this convergence, let me take you on a journey through the history of mindfulness. Mindfulness is not a new concept; in fact, its roots go back thousands of years to the ancient Buddhist traditions of India. In the "Satipatthana Sutta," an ancient Buddhist text dating back to the 5th century B.C., Gautama Buddha describes the practice of mindfulness as the only way to achieve liberation from suffering.

In recent decades, mindfulness has found its way into the Western world, thanks in large part to the work of figures such as Jon Kabat-Zinn, who in 1979 founded the Stress Reduction Clinic and the Mindfulness-Based Stress Reduction program at the University of Massachusetts. His book "Living Fully through Crises: How to Use the Wisdom of Body and Mind to Cope with Stress, Pain and Illness" (1990) has been a beacon of light for millions of people around the world.

These ancient teachings, combined with modern clinical applications of mindfulness, offer us a powerful tool for personal transformation and spiritual growth. And, as you will see in this chapter, it is this same tool that allows us to experience tantric massage at its best.

But what does it really mean to be present? What does it look like in practice? Let me explain.

To be present means to be completely immersed in what is happening at this very moment. It means that your mind is not wandering in thoughts of the past or the future, but is fully focused on what is happening now. You can be present when you eat, when you walk, when you bathe, when you read, and yes, also when you practice tantric massage.

To experience this state of mindfulness, one practice that can be very helpful is meditation. By meditating, we train ourselves in the ability to focus our mind, to keep it still and in the present, rather than allowing it to jump from one thought to another like a monkey in the jungle.

In his book "Mindfulness in Everyday Life: Wherever You Go, There You Are" (1994), Jon Kabat-Zinn explains that meditating is nothing more than paying attention in a particular way: deliberately, in the present moment and without judgment. And this is precisely the attitude we need when we practice tantric massage.

Tantric massage is a dance, a deep interaction between two bodies and two souls. It is a conversation without words, where language is touch and listening is the perception of energy and sensations. But to participate fully in this conversation, we must be present, we must pay attention.

You are probably asking yourself, how can I do that? How can I be present in tantric massage? Let me offer you some guidance.

Before you begin the massage, take a moment to focus on yourself. Close your eyes, breathe deeply and pay attention to the sensations in your body. Do you feel tension somewhere? Is there a part of your body that is asking for your attention? How does the air feel as it moves in and out of your lungs? This act of paying attention to your body, without judging, without trying to change anything, is already an act of meditation, an act of being present.

As you begin the massage, bring this same attention to your partner's hands, or your own if you are the one giving the massage. Pay attention to every caress, every touch, every change in pressure. Notice how it feels on your skin, in your muscles, in your bones. Let each caress be like the drop of water on the window, a unique and unrepeatable experience that invites you to be in the present.

This level of presence is not easy to achieve, but do not despair. Remember, mindfulness is a practice. Like a muscle, mindfulness gets stronger with time and practice. And each time you do, you are taking one more step on your path to a deeper and more enriching experience of tantric massage.

But why is this mindfulness so important in tantric massage? What happens when we are present? To answer these questions, we will explore a little more about the importance of this presence in the following section.

Imagine you are at a concert. The music is vibrant and fills the space. But instead of listening, you're on your phone, texting your friends about how exciting the concert is. Even though you're physically there, you're actually missing out on the experience. You're not really listening to the music, you're not really feeling the energy of the place. You're disconnected, absent, not present.

The same is true in tantric massage. If while you are in the session your mind is thinking about work, pending tasks or anything else, you are missing out on the experience. You are disconnected from your body, your partner and the sensations you might be experiencing.

Mindfulness, then, is like a bridge that connects us to direct experience, allowing us to fully experience each moment of tantric massage. And when we are present, something wonderful happens: we open ourselves to the possibility of a deeper pleasure, a more intimate connection and a more complete liberation.

Consider this example. Imagine you are giving a tantric massage and your mind starts to wander. You start thinking about what you are going to do next, a problem you have at work, or a worry you have. Suddenly, your hand starts moving automatically, not paying attention to the signals your partner's body is giving you. You may get out of sync with their breathing, you may not realize that a part of their body needs more attention, or you may apply too much pressure without realizing it. You are there, but at the same time you are not there.

Now, imagine that in that same massage, you realize that your mind has begun to wander. But instead of following that thought, you decide to return to your breath, to the sensations of your body, to the hands on your partner's skin. You begin to listen again, to feel again, to be present again. And in that moment, you can adjust your touch, you can tune into your partner's breathing, you can be totally there, in the massage. That's the difference that mindfulness makes.

Philosopher Alan Watts once said, "This is the eternal present. Here. Now. But most people don't recognize it. They are stuck in the past, thinking about what happened yesterday or ten years ago. Or they are worried about the future, thinking about what will happen tomorrow or next year. But the past is gone and the future has not yet arrived. All we have is the present. And the present is all there is."

And this is exactly the gift that tantric massage offers you: the opportunity to be in the present, to experience the power of the now, to fully enjoy every caress, every touch, every vibration of energy.

In summary, mindfulness and meditation are essential tools in the practice of tantric massage. They allow us to be present in the massage, to fully feel each sensation, and to establish a deeper connection with our partner and ourselves. They allow us to transform tantric massage into a true meditation in movement, a dance of awareness and pleasure.

And while these tools may seem simple, their impact is profoundly transformative. As Jon Kabat-Zinn, one of the pioneers of mindfulness meditation in the West, said, "mindfulness is the awareness that comes from paying attention, intentionally, in the present moment, and without judgment, to things as they are."

This is the consciousness you can cultivate in tantric massage. Not a fragmented, distracted awareness, lost in thoughts of the past or the future. But a full, present awareness, open to the sensations of the now.

Every breath, every touch, every caress, becomes an invitation to be fully here and now, to experience the ecstasy of the present moment. And as you cultivate this presence, you realize that each moment is unique, unrepeatable, full of possibilities.

Dear reader, the practice of mindfulness and meditation in tantric massage invites you to awaken to this reality. It invites you to live each moment of the session as if it were the only moment that exists. It invites you to discover the power of the now, the depth of the present, the dance of ecstasy.

So it is no exaggeration to say that mindfulness and meditation can transform your experience of tantric massage, and through it, your relationship with yourself and your partner. And remember, you don't need to be an expert meditator or a seasoned yogi to get started. You just need the willingness to be present, to pay attention, to open to the now.

In this chapter we have explored the fascinating world of mindfulness and meditation in tantric massage. We have discovered how these practices can deepen our connection with the body, enhance our pleasure and transform our experience of the session.

I hope you have enjoyed this journey as much as I enjoyed writing it. But this is not the end, but just the beginning. In the next chapter, we will delve into the magic of ritual in tantric massage. We will discover how to create a sacred space for the session, how to use symbols and objects to empower our intention, and how ritual can help us prepare for the session and integrate the experience afterwards.

So, are you ready to keep exploring, to keep discovering, to keep growing on this wonderful path of tantra? Are you ready to keep moving forward on this journey to the heart of tantric massage? If so, I invite you to go ahead, to open the door to the next chapter and dive back into the dance of ecstasy. I await you there.

Chapter 12: The Magic of Ritual: Creating a Sacred Space

Let me take you on a journey, dear reader. Imagine you are standing at the entrance of an ancient temple. As you approach, you can smell the scent of flowers and incense in the air, hear the echoes of mantras and sacred chants, feel the peace and serenity that permeates the atmosphere. You realize that it is not an ordinary place, it is a sacred space.

Can you feel it? That feeling of respect and reverence, of awe and wonder, of calm and serenity. You feel immersed in an atmosphere full of meaning, in a dimension where every detail, every gesture, every word, acquires a deep meaning. Wouldn't it be wonderful to be able to create such a space for your tantric massage?

In this chapter, we are going to explore the magic of ritual and how we can use it to create a sacred space for tantric massage. But before that, let me ask you a question: Why do you think it is important to create a sacred space for tantric massage practice?

The answer is simple and profound at the same time: because the space in which we perform tantric massage is not only a physical place, it is also a space of consciousness, a space of encounter, a space of transformation.

That is why it is essential to create a space that invites relaxation, presence, intimacy, surrender, exploration and enjoyment. A space that allows us to move away from the hustle and bustle and noise of the outside world, to enter into the silence and stillness of our inner world. A space that allows us to connect with ourselves, with our partner, with the present moment, with the energy of life.

In the Tantric tradition, the creation of this sacred space is an art and a science in itself. It involves the use of various symbolic elements, rituals and techniques, which help us to change our perception and deepen our experience of tantric massage. But before we get into these practical aspects, I would like to invite you to reflect on the very nature of ritual.

What is a ritual, why is it so powerful, how can it help us create sacred space?

To answer these questions, let me quote Joseph Campbell, a renowned expert in mythology and author of "The Hero with a Thousand Faces" (1949). According to Campbell, "a ritual is the performance of a myth. And, by participating in the ritual, you are participating in the myth. And since the myth is related to the fundamental structure of reality, you are participating in reality."

This idea is fundamental to understanding the magic of ritual in tantric massage. Because when we perform a ritual, we are not simply performing meaningless actions. We are participating in a myth, in a sacred story, in a journey of transformation. We are participating in reality itself, in the sacred dance of energy and consciousness, in the revelation and celebration of life in its fullness.

Now that we have a better understanding of what ritual means, let's delve into how we can create our own ritual for tantric massage. In this regard, I would like to quote Carl

Jung, the famous Swiss psychiatrist and psychologist, and one of the great thinkers of the 20th century. In his work "Man and his Symbols" (1964), Jung pointed out: "Rituals, like symbols, are as old as man himself and permeate all aspects of human life".

So how is this reflected in our tantric massage practice? Well, the first and perhaps most obvious way to incorporate ritual into tantric massage is through the creation of a conducive physical environment. This may include the careful selection of a quiet, private place, the creation of a dimly lit environment, perhaps through candles, the use of incense or essential oils to stimulate the senses, the preparation of a comfortable surface for massage, and so on.

The preparation of this physical environment is not just a matter of aesthetics or comfort, but is a way of expressing our respect and reverence for ourselves, for our partner, and for the sacred act of giving and receiving a tantric massage. Therefore, I encourage you to devote time and attention to creating your sacred space for tantric massage.

But the tantric massage ritual is not limited to the preparation of the physical space. It also includes a series of symbolic actions and gestures that help us to attune our mind and body to the energy of the present moment. This may include performing a meditation or breathing exercise at the beginning of the massage, using mantras or positive affirmations, setting an intention for the massage, performing certain movements or gestures with the hands before beginning the massage, and so on.

These symbolic actions and gestures help us connect with the energy of the present moment and deepen our experience of tantric massage. But have you ever wondered why these rituals are so powerful?

To answer this question, let me quote Mircea Eliade, a leading historian of religions and author of "The Myth of Eternal Return" (1949). According to Eliade, "a ritual opens a 'sacred today', a temporal discontinuity that allows the individual to relive the 'mythical time', the 'primordial time', the 'deep time'".

In other words, rituals allow us to connect with a dimension of reality that goes beyond ordinary time and space, a dimension where we can experience the fullness of life and the depth of our being. Therefore, I encourage you to incorporate ritual into your tantric massage practice and to explore its transformative power.

But what if you have never performed a ritual before, how can you incorporate these elements into your tantric massage practice in a meaningful way? Let me give you a practical example to illustrate this.

Imagine you are preparing to give a tantric massage to your partner. You have created a conducive physical environment: you have chosen a quiet and private place, you have created a dimly lit environment with candles, you have prepared a comfortable surface for the massage, you have used incense and essential oils to stimulate the senses.

But before starting the massage, you decide to perform a ritual to attune your mind and body to the present moment.

You sit in a comfortable position, close your eyes and begin to breathe consciously and deeply. You become aware of the sensation of the air moving in and out of your lungs, the feeling of your body in contact with the ground, the sensation of energy flowing through your body.

Then, you start repeating a mantra in your mind. The mantra can be any word or phrase that has special meaning to you, such as "Love", "Peace", "Harmony", "Oneness", "Consciousness", "Life". As you repeat the mantra, you notice that your mind becomes calmer and more centered, your body relaxes and feels more alive, your heart opens and fills with love and gratitude.

Finally, you set an intention for the massage. The intention can be anything you wish for you and your partner, such as "May this massage bring us healing and relaxation," "May this massage allow us to connect on a deeper level," "May this massage open us to the experience of ecstasy and oneness." As you set the intention, you feel a deep sense of purpose and commitment, of openness and surrender, of anticipation and joy.

This is how you could incorporate ritual into your tantric massage practice. As you can see, it's not about performing meaningless actions or following rigid rules. It is about creating a space of awareness and presence, of respect and reverence, of intention and purpose, of love and ecstasy. It is about participating in the sacred dance of life and consciousness, about revealing and celebrating the beauty and divinity that dwells within you and your partner.

Now, let me quote Ram Dass, a famous psychologist and spiritualist and author of "Here and Now: Journey to Spiritual Awakening" (1971). According to Ram Dass, "Ritual is a vehicle that transports the spirit."

So, dear reader, I invite you to use ritual as a vehicle to transport your spirit on the journey of tantric massage. I invite you to explore the magic of ritual and to create your own sacred space for tantric massage practice.

Chapter 13: The Language of the Body: Nonverbal Communication in Tantra

When you enter the world of Tantra, you encounter a new language, a language that goes beyond words. A language that is based on the subtleties of energy, emotional currents and the wisdom of the body. We are talking about body language or non-verbal communication.

You may ask, why is nonverbal communication so important in Tantra? I invite you to reflect on this. Think about your own experiences, how many times have you felt that words fail to fully express what you feel or experience? How many times have you perceived a dissonance between what someone says and how they behave? How many times have you felt a deep connection with someone, without the need to speak?

The body has its own intelligence and its own voice, a voice that expresses itself through movement, posture, breath, gaze, touch. And when we learn to listen and speak this language of the body, we can establish a deeper and more authentic connection with ourselves and with others. In the context of tantric massage, non-verbal communication is the key to tuning into your partner's energy, to responding to their needs and desires, to guiding and being guided on the journey of ecstasy.

Some of the most important elements of nonverbal communication in Tantra include sensory perception, kinesthetic empathy, intuition, presence, authenticity, and intention. We will delve into each of these aspects in this chapter.

However, before we go into these elements, it is crucial to understand that non-verbal communication in Tantra is not a technique that you can learn from a book or a course. It is not something you can "do" with your mind. It is something you have to "be" with your whole being. It is an art that requires sensitivity, receptivity, attention, patience, practice and, above all, love. Are you ready to embark on this journey of discovery and exploration?

I am not talking about learning to "read" body language in the conventional sense. I am not talking about looking for signs and clues, interpreting gestures and expressions, analyzing behaviors and reactions. This can be useful in certain contexts, but in Tantra, we are looking for something deeper and more subtle. We are looking for a soul-to-soul connection, an energetic dance, a dialogue without words, a communion of beings.

So don't worry if you're not an expert in body language. You don't need to be a detective or a psychologist. You just need to be yourself, with all your heart and all your presence. You just need to be willing to open to the experience, to feel and respond to the energy, to flow with the moment, to surrender to the ecstasy.

Are you ready to learn this new language of the body, this language of Tantra? This is a journey of discovery, of exploration and, most importantly, of deep understanding. Let's see how non-verbal communication really works in the world of Tantra.

First, let's talk about sensory perception. You have five senses: touch, sight, hearing, taste and smell. Each of these senses allows you to interact and perceive the world in different ways. But in Tantra practice, we focus primarily on touch and sight, with hearing playing a secondary role. By touching, you can perceive the subtleties of your partner's body, the tensions and relaxations, the responses and resistances, the pulses and flows of energy. Through sight, you can connect with your partner's presence, energy and soul. And through hearing, you can tune in to your partner's breath, to the subtle sounds and silences that guide you on the journey.

To illustrate this, let us recall the words of Michaela Boehm in her work "The Wild Woman's Way" (2018), where she says: "Sensation is the language of the body. It is through our sensations that we know our truth and what is real to us." In other words, it is through our sensory perception that we connect with the reality of our body and that of others.

Kinesthetic empathy is another crucial element of nonverbal communication in Tantra. Remember when you were feeling sad and a friend hugged you and somehow, even though he didn't say anything, you felt that he understood your pain? That is kinesthetic empathy. It is the ability to feel with the body what another person is feeling. In tantric massage, this kinesthetic empathy allows us to tune into our partner's sensations and emotions, to respond appropriately and authentically.

Intuition also plays an important role. Have you ever had a feeling about something and it turned out to be true? That's your intuition at play. It's an inner sense that often gets lost in the cacophony of our daily lives. But in Tantra, we make space for this intuition, allowing us to move fluidly and respond to our partner in a way that goes beyond what our physical senses can perceive.

The understanding of presence, authenticity and intention also plays a vital role. Being present does not only mean being physically in a place, but also bringing your whole attention, your whole being to that moment. It is being in the "now" and nowhere else. Authenticity is being yourself, without masks, without pretense. And intention is the driving force behind your actions, it is what drives you to act in a particular way.

As we explore each of these elements, I encourage you to remember that nonverbal communication in Tantra is an art. And like any art, it requires practice and patience. But beyond that, it requires love. Love for yourself, love for your partner and love for the shared experience.

I want to share with you an example to illustrate these concepts in a more tangible way. Imagine you are in a tantric massage session with your partner. You are fully present in the room, with every one of your senses tuned and focused on your partner. You observe the nuances of his breathing, the small movements of his body, the subtle sounds he makes. You see the micro-expressions on his face and feel the energy flowing between you. Now, as you do all this, you are also in a state of total authenticity. You are not trying to be someone you are not, you are simply surrendering to the experience, trusting your intuition and the power of your intention to bring pleasure and healing.

As the session progresses, you notice a slight tension in your partner's shoulders. You can see it, you can feel it under your hands. Instead of ignoring it, you allow your kinesthetic empathy to activate. You feel the tension in your own body, an echo of hers. And then, with love and care, you focus your energy on that area, massaging it, releasing the tension until you feel your partner's body relax once again. This, my friend, is nonverbal communication in action.

It is a language without words, an exchange of energies and emotions that allow you to tune into your partner's rhythm in a way that words often cannot capture. It allows you to listen, not just with your ears, but with your whole being. And in doing so, you connect with your partner on a deeply intimate level.

In her book "Tantric Orgasm for Women" (2004), author Diana Richardson explains: "Tantra is the art of being present, which involves allowing ourselves to be who we are in this moment, accepting ourselves as we are". It is in that acceptance that we find the freedom to connect with others in an authentic and meaningful way.

Here I pause, and ask you, can you recall an occasion when you have communicated without words? A look, a touch, a sigh that spoke volumes? How did that make you feel?

Communicating without words is not only an essential skill in Tantra, but in all aspects of our lives. It allows us to connect more deeply and meaningfully with the people around us, and helps us to understand and empathize with their experiences.

The practice of Tantra is, in essence, a dance of energy. And just as in any dance, we need to learn to listen to ourselves and respond to our fellow dancers. Nonverbal communication is the key to doing just that. By perfecting this form of communication, we not only enhance our Tantra practice, but we also open ourselves to new forms of connection and understanding.

But remember, nonverbal communication is not a one-way street. As you learn to read your partner's nonverbal signals, it is equally important that you learn to convey your own. As Margot Anand says in her work "The Art of Sexual Ecstasy" (1989), "Tantra is an invitation to experience the fullness and depth of our own energies and emotions, and to express them authentically and courageously." It is a call to be seen, felt and understood.

Every time you show your emotions, your needs, your pleasure and your love through your body language, you are honoring your truth and allowing others to connect with you in a deeper way.

Imagine a world where we all learn to communicate in this way. Where authenticity, empathy and respect form the basis of our interactions. A world where we learn to listen to each other, to really listen to each other, with our whole selves. Sounds amazing, doesn't it? And it is within your reach, dear reader, because it starts with you, with your choice to learn this beautiful language of the body and the heart.

I must emphasize that the road to effective nonverbal communication is not always easy. It requires patience, practice, and sometimes a willingness to face our own insecurities and fears. But I promise you it's worth it. Because once you begin to understand and speak this language without words, you will open the door to a dimension of connection and understanding that surpasses the limits of verbal communication.

In this chapter, we have navigated together through the importance and depth of nonverbal communication in the practice of Tantra. We have explored how our ability to listen, feel and respond to nonverbal cues can enhance our relationships and our understanding of ourselves and others. And, most importantly, I have invited you to immerse yourself in the universe of nonverbal communication and discover for yourself the power and beauty of this wordless language.

It is my sincere hope that this chapter has inspired you to further explore nonverbal communication in your own tantric path. I invite you to take with you the ideas and practices we have discussed, and integrate them into your daily practice. And remember, as always, practice makes perfect.

If you are ready to continue on this path of discovery and transformation, I look forward to seeing you in the next chapter. There, we will explore how Tantra can be a powerful tool for emotional healing. We'll discover how conscious, loving touch can help release old traumas and open us to new possibilities for love, connection and joy.

I feel a tingle of anticipation as we prepare to take the next step in our journey. Do you feel it too? Are you ready to further explore the mysteries of Tantra and to unleash the healing power of touch? Then join me, dear friend, and let's take that step together.

Chapter 14: Healing Through Touch: Tantric Massage and Emotional Health

Have you ever felt how a simple hug can comfort you in times of sadness? Have you experienced the relief of a gentle shoulder massage after a stressful day? Have you noticed how your heart seems to melt when someone you love holds your hand in a time of need? All this is no accident, my friend.

Touch has an extraordinary healing power, one that we often underestimate in our society obsessed with words and rational explanations. But what if we could learn to touch in a way that conveyed love, acceptance and compassion, that could help heal old wounds and release emotional blockages? What if Tantric massage, a practice that combines the power of conscious touch with the spiritual teachings of Tantra, were a doorway to that possibility?

Let's talk about it.

Tantric massage, as you know from the previous chapters, is much more than a massage technique. It is a spiritual practice, a path to self-awareness and personal transformation. It is a form of communication, a language of the body that transcends words. But it is also, and this is what we are concerned with in this chapter, a powerful tool for emotional health.

Why is this so important?

Because we all carry emotional scars. Some are obvious, like the pain of a loss or a betrayal. Others are hidden, such as forgotten childhood traumas or limiting beliefs we have internalized over the years. But they all affect the way we relate to ourselves, to others and to the world. They can make us feel disconnected, alone, trapped in patterns of thought and behavior that cause us suffering.

This is where tantric massage comes in. By using conscious touch, we can reach these emotional wounds in a way that words often cannot. We can offer comfort and understanding, we can help release the emotional tension stored in the body, we can open a space for the person to feel seen, accepted and loved.

But how exactly does this work? How can a simple touch reach deep into our psyche and promote emotional healing? And how can you learn to touch in this way yourself?

I invite you to join me on this journey of exploration. Together, we will delve into the secrets of healing touch, discover how tantric massage can help us release old traumas and open us to new possibilities of love, connection and joy.

Are you ready to get started?

Here we go!

Now, my friend, think for a moment about how you feel when you touch yourself. I'm not talking about a casual caress or an automatic gesture, but a conscious and present touch. Maybe you place your hand on your chest when you feel excited, or you massage your temples when you're stressed. Maybe you rub your hands together when you're nervous or stroke your arm when you're sad. Have you ever stopped to think about why you do this?

In our culture, we are often taught to repress our emotions, to be strong and to "keep our composure." But our body has an inherent wisdom, an intuitive ability to seek comfort and relief through touch. And often, when we allow ourselves this simple gesture of self-comfort, we find a profound sense of calm and relief. Have you noticed this?

This is the power of conscious touch, a power that we all carry within us and that we can learn to use in a more intentional and healing way. And it is not limited to self-healing, we can also extend it to others, through tantric massage.

Modern psychology and neuroscience give us some clues as to how this works. For example, touch therapist and author Phyllis Davis, in her book "Touch Therapy" (2002), explains that touch can help regulate our nervous system, relieve stress and increase the production of hormones such as oxytocin, often called the "love hormone".

Other studies, such as the one conducted by psychologist Tiffany Field and her colleagues at the University of Miami's Touch Research Institute, have shown that touch can help reduce pain, improve mood, and even strengthen the immune system.

And while this research does not focus specifically on tantric massage, it provides a scientific framework that helps us understand how this practice can promote emotional health.

But beyond the physiological mechanisms, there is the spiritual and emotional dimension of conscious touch. In his book "The Body Keeps the Score" (2014), psychiatrist Bessel van der Kolk tells us how traumas can become "imprinted" on our bodies, and how techniques involving the body and touch, such as tantric massage, can help release these traumas and promote healing.

Tantric massage offers us a way of touching and being touched that goes beyond the purely physical. It allows us to communicate and receive love, compassion, and acceptance. It allows us to reconnect with our body and our emotions, and to open ourselves to experiences of deep intimacy and connection.

So, you see, tantric massage is not just a technique. It is a practice that takes us on a journey to the heart of our humanity, to a place of deep empathy and compassion. A place where we can heal and be healed. And, on this journey, we also learn to heal others, to touch others in a way that honors and celebrates their humanity, their vulnerability, and their divinity. Isn't this beautiful, my friend?

Now, you may be wondering, how does all this translate into practice? What does a tantric massage that promotes emotional health look and feel like?

I'll tell you one thing, it's not that different from any other form of massage as far as technique is concerned. But as far as intention and presence, it's a world apart.

Imagine you are giving a tantric massage to your partner. You are both naked, in a space you have prepared together, filled with soft light, pleasant fragrances, and relaxing music. You have spent the last few minutes focusing on your breath, tuning into your body, and connecting with a sense of love and compassion.

Then, with the utmost care and reverence, you begin to touch your partner's body. But it is not an automatic, impersonal touch. It is a touch that says, "I see you. I honor you. I am here for you." A touch that is fully present, fully focused on the here and now.

As your hands move over your partner's body, you are aware of every sensation, every response. You watch as she tenses or relaxes under your hands. You feel how their breathing changes, how their body opens or closes to your touch.

And at all times, you are there, present, connected, loving. There is no rush. There is no goal. Just the sacred act of touching and being touched.

But a tantric massage is also a dialogue, a nonverbal communication that we explored in chapter 13. And just as in any dialogue, it is important to listen. So, you listen. You listen with your hands, with your body. You listen to the signals your partner's body gives you. And you respond to them, adjusting your touch, your pressure, your rhythm, according to what you feel your partner needs and wants at that moment.

So, a tantric massage is, in essence, a practice of mindfulness, presence and love. And through this practice, we can open a healing space, a space where both the giver and receiver can explore and release emotions, traumas, and blockages that may be stored in their body.

I could give you more examples, but I think this one gives you an idea of what it means to give and receive a tantric massage. And I assure you, there is nothing like direct experience.

So why not give it a try? In the next chapter, I will guide you through some tantric massage techniques and sequences that you can practice. But for now, I simply invite you to reflect on what we have discussed in this chapter. And, perhaps, to explore a bit for yourself. After all, the path to the heart of tantric massage always begins with a single step.

Look, the truth is that sometimes we can feel a little intimidated when starting something new, especially something as intimate and deep as tantric massage. But I assure you, my friend, there is nothing to be afraid of. On the contrary, there is so much to discover, so much to explore, so much to enjoy.....

You don't have to be an expert, you don't need to have previous experience. All you need is a heart willing to learn and open, and a body willing to feel and let go. And, of course, a little guidance, which is precisely what I will offer you in the next chapter.

In Chapter 15, I will go into more detail about the specific techniques and sequences you can use in tantric massage. I will show you how you can use your hands, your fingers, your whole body, to touch and move energy in ways that can lead to healing and ecstasy. I will show you how you can create a safe and sacred space for your practice, how you can communicate with your partner so that the experience is rewarding for both of you, and how you can take care of yourself so that you can continue to give and receive with joy and love.

And most importantly, I will remind you again and again that tantric massage is not so much about technique, but about presence, attention, intention. Because ultimately, what heals and transforms is not the touch itself, but the love and compassion with which you touch.

So, are you ready to move forward? Are you ready to embark on this wonderful journey of self-discovery and growth? Are you ready to experience the magic of tantric massage for yourself?

I promise you it will be worth it, not only for the pleasure and joy it can bring to your life, but also for the profound healing and transformation it can facilitate. And remember, I am always here for you, accompanying you every step of the way.

Therefore, I encourage you to move forward with courage, with curiosity, with openness. Let anticipation fill you with excitement, but also let peace wrap you in its warm embrace. Because you are about to enter a space of love, of healing, of growth. A space where you can be yourself, where you can be vulnerable, where you can be authentically human.

And always remember, the real journey is not outward, but inward. So go on, move forward. I look forward to seeing you in the next chapter. See you there, my friend.

Chapter 15: Tantric Massage Techniques and Sequences: A Journey through the Body

Have you ever wondered why hugs feel so good? Why, when we are sad, distressed or just in need of comfort, human touch has such a calming and healing effect? Have you ever thought about how touch can communicate so many things, from love and tenderness to desire and passion?

That is the magic of touch, and that is the power of tantric massage. Because tantric massage is not simply a series of movements and techniques; it is a way of communication, a way of connecting, a way of touching and being touched that goes far beyond the skin.

Why is it important to learn tantric massage techniques and sequences? Is it not enough to let oneself be carried away by intuition, by love, by desire?

While it is true that intuition, love and desire are fundamental components of tantric massage, it is also true that knowledge and practice of certain techniques and sequences can enhance and enrich the experience. They will allow you to move and manipulate energy in more efficient and effective ways, help you avoid possible injury or discomfort, and give you greater confidence and skill in your interactions.

Think of it this way: if you are learning to play a musical instrument, isn't it useful to know the notes, the chords, the scales? Isn't it useful to learn how to hold the instrument, how to move your hands, how to breathe? The same goes for tantric massage. By learning the techniques and sequences, you are learning the language of touch, you are learning how to play the most wonderful and complex instrument of all: the human body.

And so, as when you play music, it is not just about the notes you play, but how you play them, the intention and emotion you put into each movement, each gesture. So as I teach you these techniques and sequences, I will always remind you that the heart of tantric massage is not in the hands, but in the heart.

Throughout this chapter, I will guide you through various aspects of tantric massage, including preparation for the massage, touch techniques, the massage sequence, and how to handle any emotions or energies that may arise during the massage. I'll give you practical tools and tips that you can start using immediately. And, of course, I will show you how all of this connects and intertwines with what we have already covered in the previous chapters.

So, are you ready to embark on this fascinating journey through the body? Are you ready to discover new ways to touch, to connect, to love? Because, I promise you, what you will learn in this chapter will surprise and amaze you. And not only that, it will profoundly change the way you experience and understand human touch, love and desire. Because, after all, that's what tantric massage, at its core, is all about: expanding our perceptions, challenging our limitations, awakening to a new way of being and relating.

You may already be familiar with some of the tantric massage techniques we will explore here. Some of them are based on ancient practices, which have been passed down from generation to generation, from teacher to student, from lover to lover. Others come from modern disciplines, such as physical therapy, osteopathy and chiropractic, which have studied the human body with a scientific and medical approach.

For example, the "breath awareness" technique taught in many tantric traditions has striking parallels with diaphragmatic breathing techniques used in physical therapy to improve lung capacity, circulation and relaxation. Similarly, "energetic pulsation," which is used in tantric massage to move and release energy, has much in common with joint mobilization techniques used in osteopathy and chiropractic.

In fact, the famous British osteopath and physiotherapist, Leon Chaitow, in his book "Soft Tissue Manipulation: A Practitioner's Guide to the Diagnosis and Treatment of Soft Tissue Dysfunction and Reflex Activity" (1980), explains how soft tissue manipulation techniques, when applied correctly, can have profound effects on the nervous system and the release of repressed emotions, a statement that aligns perfectly with the teachings of tantra.

Another tantric technique you might find familiar is "energy polarization," which is a way of playing and experimenting with the masculine and feminine energies in the body. This technique has echoes of the theory of polarity, developed by Dr. Randolph Stone in the 1940s, which also speaks to the importance of balancing masculine and feminine energies for health and well-being.

But tantric massage is not just a collection of techniques and theories from different disciplines. It has its own philosophy and its own principles, which are based on the tantric understanding of energy and consciousness. So, while I introduce you to these techniques and sequences, I will also tell you about the tantric vision that underlies them, how every movement, every gesture, every touch can be a form of meditation, a form of worship, a form of union.

Because, remember, tantric massage is not only a physical practice, it is a spiritual practice. It is a way of touching the body to reach the soul. It is a way to awaken the energy to reach the consciousness. It is a way to celebrate and honor life in all its dimensions and expressions.

So, let me take you on a journey, a journey through the hills and valleys of your body, a journey through the currents and tides of your energy, a journey through the secrets and mysteries of your being. And, as we travel together, I will show you how each stop on this journey, each tantric massage technique and sequence, can be a doorway to a new world of insights and experiences.

We will begin with "massage preparation", which is an often overlooked but crucial aspect of tantric massage. I will teach you how to cleanse and energize your space, how to attune and warm your body, how to invoke and channel your intention. At this point, you may remember Chapter 12, where we talked about "The Magic of Ritual: Creating Sacred Space." Now let's take those concepts to a more practical and tangible level.

Then we will move on to "touch techniques", where I will show you how your hands can become instruments of love and healing. I will teach you to play with awareness and presence, to play with sensitivity and respect, to play with passion and tenderness. You will learn to vary pressure and speed, to use different parts of your hands, to follow and guide the breath. I will teach you to "listen" with your hands, to tune in to the subtle signals of the body and energy. Here, you may recall chapter 2, where we explored "The Alchemy of Touch: From Skin to Soul", and you will realize how what we are learning now is rooted in what you have learned before.

Then we will go into the "massage sequence", where you will learn to move and flow through the body like a dancer, like a musician, like a poet. I will teach you to create a rhythm and a flow, to move from one area of the body to another, to mix different techniques and styles. You will learn how to work with the chakras, those energy centers we discussed in chapter 10, and how each chakra can be stimulated and balanced through massage.

Finally, we will address the management of "energy and emotions" that may arise during the massage. I will give you tips and tools for handling arousal, release, vulnerability, intimacy. I will show you how tantric massage can be a safe space to explore and express your emotions and desires, and how it can be a powerful tool for healing and transformation. If you think back to Chapter 14, where we discussed "Healing Through Touch: Tantric Massage and Emotional Health," you will realize how this aspect of tantric massage aligns with that understanding.

Now, let me give you a concrete example of how all this can be integrated into a tantric massage session.

Imagine that you are preparing the space for the massage. Clean the room, light some candles, put on some soft music. Make sure the temperature is comfortable and that there are enough pillows and blankets. Then, take a moment to tune into yourself, to breathe deeply and set your intention. You may wish to repeat quietly or in your mind something like, "My intention is to play with love, respect and awareness."

Now imagine that your partner is lying in front of you, her body naked and vulnerable, fully trusting you. Start by gently touching her feet, then slowly move up her legs, her thighs, her pelvis. Remember to vary the pressure and speed, remember to follow and guide her breathing. Watch how her body responds to your touch, how her energy flows and changes.

Then, he continues with the torso, the arms, the neck. Finally reach the face, gently touch her cheeks, her lips, her forehead. As you do this, keep your mind and heart open, keep your attention on the present, on each sensation, on each emotion.

Perhaps at some point you will feel an intense emotion or powerful energy emerging, perhaps you will see tears in their eyes or hear a deep sigh. In that moment, breathe with him, hold your presence and your compassion, remember that you are providing a safe space for his expression and release.

Finally, close the massage with a sequence of soft and slow touches, like a lullaby for his body and soul. Then, allow him to rest, allow him to integrate all that he has experienced. In the meantime, be silently grateful for the opportunity to share this journey, to touch and be touched, to love and be loved.

Do you see how tantric massage can be much more than just a set of techniques and sequences? Do you see how it can be a path of connection and transformation, of love and ecstasy? In its essence, tantric massage is an art, it is a dance, it is a meditation, it is a prayer.

We have journeyed together throughout this chapter, exploring the wonders of tantric massage. We have learned about massage preparation, touch techniques, massage sequencing, and the management of energy and emotions. We have seen how each of these aspects is important and how they intertwine to create a profound and transformative experience.

In our next chapter, we will delve into a fascinating and powerful concept, the "Synthesis of Opposites: Integration and Balance." We will explore how tantric massage can help us integrate and balance our inner polarities, our lights and shadows, our masculine and feminine selves.

Chapter 16: The Synthesis of Opposites: Integration and Equilibrium

Have you ever felt that you have two contradictory parts inside you, fighting against each other? Have you ever wished you could integrate these parts and find a balance? If so, you are in the right place.

Tantra teachings tell us that we all carry within us a sun and a moon, a yin and a yang, a masculine and a feminine energy. These energies have nothing to do with our physical gender, they are universal energies that we all carry within us, regardless of whether we are male or female. In the tantric tradition, these energies are considered complementary, not opposites. Each has its own qualities and functions, and both are necessary for our health and well-being.

The masculine energy, also known as Shiva, is associated with consciousness, presence, stability, direction. It is the sky, it is the mountain, it is the fire that illuminates and warms. The feminine energy, also known as Shakti, is associated with energy, creativity, sensitivity, movement. It is the earth, it is the river, it is the water that nourishes and purifies.

When these energies are in balance, we feel complete, whole, at peace. Our mind is clear, our body is vibrant, our heart is open. But when these energies are out of balance, we can feel confused, unstable, unsatisfied. We may feel as if we are fighting against ourselves, as if we are trying to fill a void we cannot name.

This is where tantric massage comes in. Through its integral and holistic approach, tantric massage helps us to balance and synthesize our inner energies, to integrate our polarities and to embrace our wholeness. Instead of judging or repressing our inner contradictions, tantric massage invites us to accept them, to explore them, to dance with them.

So I invite you to join me on this journey of integration and balance, of synthesis and union. I invite you to discover how tantric massage can help you to reconcile with yourself, to find peace within yourself, to experience the ecstasy of being fully you.

Are you ready to embark on this journey of self-discovery and transformation? Are you ready to unlock the unlimited potential within you? Then let's take the first step together on this path of integration and balance, of synthesis of opposites.

In the following section, we will explore some profound teachings and practices that will help you understand and balance your inner energies, integrate your polarities and live from a place of wholeness and harmony. I will share with you some secrets and techniques from the ancient tantric traditions that have been passed down from generation to generation, through teachers and disciples, since the dawn of civilization.

Carl Jung, one of the most influential psychologists of the 20th century, talked about these complementary energies in his works. In his book "Archetypes and the Collective Unconscious" (1959), he mentioned that every individual has a feminine and a masculine aspect, which he called anima and animus, respectively. Jung believed that to achieve true wholeness, a person must recognize and balance these two energies within himself.

The most interesting thing is that this idea of integrating opposites is not only theoretical, but can be lived in a practical and tangible way. I propose an exercise: close your eyes for a moment and imagine that you are on top of a mountain. You can feel the firmness and stability of the rock under your feet, the fresh, clean air filling your lungs. This is the energy of Shiva, the masculine energy, providing structure, clarity and direction.

Now, imagine you are in the middle of a rushing river. You can feel the flow of the water around you, the constant and changing rhythm of the current. This is the energy of Shakti, the feminine energy, bringing movement, sensitivity and creativity. Can you feel the difference between these two energies? Can you feel how both are essential to your well-being and fulfillment?

Do you realize how, even in everyday life, we are constantly dancing between these two energies? When we are working on a project, we need Shiva energy to keep us focused and directed. But we also need Shakti energy to keep us flexible and open to new ideas.

In the next part, we will delve more deeply into how to integrate and balance these energies through tantric massage. I will teach you some powerful techniques that you can use to harmonize your inner energies and experience a greater level of well-being and fulfillment. Remember, we are on this journey together. You are my traveling companion on this path of discovery and transformation, and I am here to support you every step of the way. So, are you ready to continue?

Of course, integrating and balancing these opposites is no easy task. It requires time, patience and above all, a deep understanding of oneself. But don't worry, together we will take the necessary steps on this path.

As explained by Joseph Campbell, a famous mythologist, writer and teacher, in his work "The Hero with a Thousand Faces" (1949), we are all on a "hero's quest" throughout our lives, a quest for balance and wholeness. At this stage of our tantric journey, that quest leads us to the synthesis of opposites, to the integration and balance of Shiva and Shakti within us.

Now, how do we achieve this through tantric massage? Let me introduce you to a technique. Imagine you are beginning a tantric massage session. You have created a sacred space, you have set an intention and you have begun to breathe deeply, synchronizing your breathing with your partner. Now, as you apply the massage techniques we have discussed in previous chapters, begin to visualize the energies of Shiva and Shakti within you.

As you inhale, imagine the energy of Shiva ascending from the base of your spine to the center of your forehead, the third eye. As you exhale, imagine Shakti energy descending from the center of your forehead to the base of your spine. As you continue this breathing cycle, imagine these two energies meeting and intertwining at the center of your heart, creating a whirlwind of energy.

This exercise, which is a variation of kundalini meditation, will allow you to experience the synthesis of opposites in a very real and tangible way. It will help you to feel the union of the masculine and feminine energies within you, promoting greater integration and balance.

I invite you to try this exercise during your next tantric massage session. Notice how you feel before and after. Do you notice any changes in your mood, in your energy level, in your sense of well-being?

Remember that this is not a race. It's about enjoying the journey, exploring, discovering, growing. If at any point you feel lost or confused, you can always come back to this book, to this chapter, to our conversations. I am here for you, to support you every step of the way.

Are you ready to further explore this integration and balance? Ready to dive into the synthesis of opposites? Let's continue our journey, my friend. Your tantric adventure awaits.

In the ancient tantric text "Vijnanabhairava Tantra", more than one hundred techniques for achieving the synthesis of opposites are described. Some of these techniques involve meditation, breathing and, of course, tantric massage. Integration and balance are not simply philosophical concepts; they are deeply personal experiences that each of us can explore in our daily lives. And I promise you, the journey is worth it.

Remember when we talked about the energies of Shiva and Shakti in the previous chapters? We mentioned how Shiva, the masculine principle, represents pure consciousness, while

Shakti, the feminine principle, symbolizes the creative energy of the universe. How does it feel to remember that moment? Do you feel the buzz of revelations, the excitement of discoveries?

These two opposites are found in each of us, regardless of our gender. And when we allow these energies to meet, unite and merge within us, we can experience a sense of wholeness, of unity, of integration.

The light of consciousness and the joy of life meet, dancing together in the great theater of your being" - this is what Anodea Judith, the famous psychologist and author of "Wheels of Life" (1987) wrote, and I think her words beautifully capture the essence of what we are trying to achieve here.

You have come a long way on your tantric journey, and there is still much to explore. The next chapter, "The Ascending Spiral: Transcending Time and Space," will take you even further on your journey of self-discovery and transformation. Here, we will delve into how tantric massage can help you transcend physical and temporal limitations and experience a greater connection to universal energy.

I can't wait to embark on this next chapter of the journey with you. Are you ready to continue? I am sure you are in for an amazing adventure. Remember, in every step, in every breath, in every touch, there is an opportunity for growth, for transformation, for integration and balance. So take a deep breath, open your heart and get ready for the journey of a lifetime.

Together, we will explore the ecstasy of tantra and discover the beauty that lies in the synthesis of opposites. See you in the next chapter, my friend.

Chapter 17: The Ascending Spiral: Transcending Time and Space

Join me, if you will, on a journey beyond the conventional dimensions of your life. Imagine being able to shed the restrictions of time and space that seem to govern your existence. Are you intrigued? I hear you, it's a concept that may seem a bit mysterious. But I assure you, my friend, that the path of tantra can take you on this extraordinary journey.

Remember that feeling of awe and wonder when, as a child, you looked up at the starry sky on a clear night? You felt a kind of tingling in your stomach at the vastness of the universe? In those moments, time and space seemed to expand, didn't it? Well, that awe, that wonder, is an indication of what tantra can awaken in you.

The concept of transcending time and space may sound abstract, even unattainable. But haven't you already experienced moments when time seemed to stand still? Maybe it was during a hug with someone you love, or watching a particularly breathtaking sunset, or perhaps during a deep meditation. Those are the moments when you step into eternal time, a time that is not governed by clocks and timetables.

But what does it really mean to transcend time and space? In his book "The Power of Now" (1997), author Eckhart Tolle describes this state as the experience of absolute presence, the "now". It is a state in which you cease to identify with the past and the future, and become fully immersed in the present moment.

Through tantric massage and the tantric practices we have explored in the previous chapters, you can cultivate this presence and open yourself to a wider dimension of consciousness. In this state, time and space fade away, and you find yourself in a place of pure awareness, of pure presence. You become the upward spiral, ever moving, ever changing, ever expanding.

So let me ask you, are you ready to explore this new territory? Are you ready to climb aboard this tantric spaceship and embark on a journey to the stars? If the answer is yes, then prepare your heart and open your mind, because we are in for an exciting adventure.

And as we move forward on this journey, I invite you to consider that you are not alone on this tantric spaceship. In each of us, there is a life force, an energy, that yearns to connect with something greater. This energy, which ancient tantra practitioners called kundalini, is often represented as a serpent coiled at the base of the spine. When you awaken kundalini, as I taught you in Chapter 6, this energy ascends up the spine toward the skull, binding the chakras together in a powerful flow of energy. It is as if you are taking off, moving away from the gravitational field of conventional time and space constraints.

Quantum physics, in fact, supports this idea of a reality beyond time and space. Theoretical physicist John Wheeler, in his work in the 1960s, introduced the idea of "quantum foam," suggesting that at the most fundamental level, reality is a kind of energetic dance where space and time are not constant, but fluctuate. In his book "The Universe in a Nutshell" (2001), Stephen Hawking explores this idea further, suggesting that at the quantum level, time and space are malleable.

Now, you may be wondering: How does all this apply to tantra and tantric massage? Well, my friend, think of tantric massage as a means to tune into this energetic dance. As you learn to channel and move your sexual energy, as we have discussed in the previous chapters, you become more aware of this quantum dance. You begin to feel that you are not only in the universe, but that you are an integral part of it.

Remember the metaphor of the upward spiral I mentioned earlier. Like the spiral, each of us is a unique and dynamic manifestation of the universe, constantly changing and evolving. In each moment, we have the opportunity to align ourselves with this cosmic energy and allow it to guide us on our journey. Isn't it exciting to think that each of us has this potential within ourselves?

Tantra invites us to transcend the linear perception of time and the limited perception of space, and to enter into the energetic dance of the universe. It invites us to be the ascending spiral. And in this dance, each of us can find a deeper connection with ourselves, with others, and with the universe itself.

But don't believe me just because I say so. Explore it for yourself. Do you feel ready to take the next step on this journey? Are you ready to join the dance of the universe? In the next segment of this chapter, we'll delve even deeper into how you can do just that.

And here we are, dear reader, in the midst of this fascinating universe, which dances to the rhythm of its own melody. Let me tell you a little story to illustrate this a little more.

Imagine for a moment a couple of dancers, twirling and swaying to the rhythm of a soft and evocative melody. Yes, exactly, visualize how they move around the dance floor, so synchronized that they seem to be a single entity. Now, imagine that these two dancers are like you and the universe. The music, of course, is the energy that flows through everything.

At first, you may feel a little clumsy, trying to keep up with the steps and rhythm. You might step on your partner's feet or trip over your own feet. But don't worry, we've all been there. It's normal at first, just as it is when you start practicing tantra.

However, as you relax and let yourself be carried away by the music, you begin to feel the flow. You begin to anticipate your partner's movements, to understand the subtleties of the melody. You don't think about your steps, you simply feel them. You are present, you are here and now, and not in the past or in the future. You have transcended time and space, and you have merged with the dance. Can you feel it?

That is exactly what happens when you practice tantric massage. Dr. Jonn Mumford, in his book "Ecstasy Through Tantra" (1988), describes it as "the dance of ecstasy." As you channel your kundalini energy and synchronize with your partner, you are immersed in a dance of love and acceptance, of giving and receiving. You are in a state of flow, similar to how dancers move to music.

But what happens when one of the dancers decides to stop and break the dance? What happens when there is no flow, when there is resistance or fear? That is precisely the question we will explore in the next section.

Let's continue with our dance, dear reader. Now, remember the question we asked earlier, what happens when one of the dancers stops and breaks the dance?

The answer is both simple and complex. The flow is broken, the harmony is disturbed and the dance stops. However, does that mean that the music has stopped playing? No, of course not. The music, or in this case, the energy of the universe, continues to flow. But when you resist, when you stop, you disconnect yourself from that flow.

In the practice of tantra, when you resist, you are resisting yourself, your essence. You are not allowing the energy to flow through you. And that can lead to energy blockages, frustration and discontent.

But don't worry, all is not lost. Remember, we are evolving human beings. The mere fact that you become aware of your resistance is already a step in the right direction. And with practice and patience, you can learn to let go of that resistance and get back into the flow.

The famous poet and mystic Rumi wrote: "Do not be satisfied with stories, how things have gone with others. Unfold your own myth" (The Essential Teachings of Rumi, 1995). Tantra invites you to unfold your own myth, to embrace your own dance, to transcend the limitations of time and space and merge with the flow of the universe.

We've come a long way, haven't we? From the ancient origins of tantric massage to integration and balance, we've explored how tantra can transform your life and take you to new heights of awareness and ecstasy.

But wait, there's more. Are you ready for the next chapter? Are you ready to explore how tantra can deepen your relationships and create a deeper bond? I promise it will be an exciting journey, full of discoveries and revelations. So, are you ready to take the next step in this fascinating journey? I'll be waiting for you in the next chapter, dear reader - come on, you can't miss it!

Chapter 18: Tantra and Relationships: Creating a Deeper Bond

Relationships are complex, multifaceted and sometimes a real challenge, aren't they? But think for a moment, isn't it through them that we discover ourselves, learn, grow and become more complete? Relationships are mirrors that reflect our hidden parts, our fears, our hopes and our deepest desires.

Now, imagine for a moment if you could take your relationships to a whole new level, if you could create a deeper connection, a connection that goes beyond the physical and into the emotional, the energetic and the spiritual. What would that look like? And more importantly, what effect would that have on you and your life?

In this chapter, we will explore how tantra can help you do just that.

First, let's consider why this is such a valuable exploration. In our society, there is an unquenchable thirst for deep and meaningful connections. Despite being more connected than ever before thanks to technology, many people feel more isolated and disconnected than ever before. Studies show that a lack of social connection can have serious effects on our mental and physical health. On the other hand, healthy, deep relationships can increase our happiness, improve our health and lengthen our lives.

On a spiritual level, relationships are a path to personal evolution. Through them, we have the opportunity to learn about ourselves, to grow and to experience life in all its facets.

As philosopher and writer Jiddu Krishnamurti says in "The First and Ultimate Freedom" (1954), "Relationship is a mirror in which you see yourself as you are". Through relationship, you can know your fears, your desires, your judgments, and your patterns of behavior.

So how can tantra help create a deeper bond in relationships? The answer lies in the very essence of tantra: union. Tantra teaches us to see the other person as a reflection of ourselves, to transcend the I and the thou and to experience oneness. It teaches us to be fully present, to open ourselves, to be vulnerable and to accept both our lights and our shadows.

But don't be fooled, this road is not always easy. It can be uncomfortable, it can be challenging, and it can take you to places you didn't expect. But if you open yourself to it, if you give yourself to it, the fruits it can offer you are immense.

Start by asking yourself: Am I willing to explore? Am I willing to open up, to be vulnerable, to accept and love all parts of myself and each other? Am I willing to transcend my fears and step into the unknown territory of love and deep connection?

Remember, my friend, the only constant in life is change, and every change, every growth, begins with a decision. And every change, every growth, begins with a decision. Are you willing to make that decision now?

To delve deeper into how tantra can enrich our relationships, we can draw on the wisdom of several authors who have dedicated their lives to exploring and understanding love, intimacy and sacred sexuality.

John Welwood, in his book Journey of the Heart: The Way of Conscious Love (1990), argues that true intimacy in a relationship arises from the courage to open fully to ourselves and to each other, to face and accept our vulnerabilities and our shadows. In her words, "intimate relationship is the art of dancing in fire." Tantra is that fire and it is also dance. It invites us to dance with our shadows, to transform our fears and to find beauty and divinity in every moment of the relationship.

Margot Anand, one of the most renowned tantra teachers, addresses this topic in her book "The Art of Sexual Ecstasy" (1990). She stresses that tantra not only enhances our sex life, but can also help us cultivate deeper connection, more authentic communication and greater love in our relationships. In her words, "when two bodies come together in the act of love, they become a microcosm reflecting the macrocosm." That means that through our relationships, we can experience the wholeness of the universe.

But how does this translate into real life? How can we integrate tantra into our daily relationships?

First, we can begin by cultivating presence. How many times do you find yourself thinking about something else while your partner is talking to you? How many times are you physically present, but mentally you are somewhere else? Tantra invites us to be fully present, to listen not only with our ears, but with our whole body and heart.

Another key is communication. And no, we are not talking about that superficial communication where we talk about the weather or what we ate for lunch. We are talking about authentic communication, where we share our fears, our hopes, our desires and our dreams. This kind of communication takes courage, because it means being vulnerable, but it is the path to a deeper connection.

Finally, tantra invites us to see sexuality in a whole new way. It is not just about physical pleasure, although that is an important part of it. It is about the union of energies, the celebration of life and love, and the expression of our divine essence.

So, my friend, I invite you to embark on this journey. A journey to a deeper connection, a greater love and a fuller life. But remember, this journey is not a destination, it is a process, a dance, a song that unfolds with every step you take. So, are you ready to dance?

Now that we've explored the theory, it's time to dive into practical examples. Imagine, for a moment, a relationship in which every encounter is a sacred ritual, every glance an exchange of energy and every embrace an embrace of the entire universe. Can you feel the depth of that connection? Can you taste the nectar of that love?

Let me take you through an imaginary journey. Imagine you are at home with your partner. The day has been long and you're both exhausted. But, instead of falling into the routine of dinner and TV, you decide to create a space to connect. You turn off your cell phones, light candles, take a bath together and share a cup of tea. In that moment, there is nothing more important in the world than each other's presence. There are no goals to achieve, no problems to solve. It's just the two of you, sharing that sacred space.

Later, they decide to have a tantric massage. But it is not just any massage. Every caress is a gesture of love, every sigh is an expression of pleasure. And as their bodies merge into one, they realize that they are not two separate individuals, but a single energy, dancing in the eternity of the universe.

This, dear reader, is just a small sample of how tantra can transform our relationships. But don't just take the words for granted. I invite you to experience it for yourself. As Osho, a famous mystic and spiritual master, said in his book "Tantra: The Supreme Understanding" (1975), "Tantra is not a theory, it is an experience".

You may feel fear. That is normal. We're talking about opening up in a way we may never have experienced before. But remember, fear is simply resistance to change. And change, while it can be challenging at times, is the path to growth and transformation.

So I invite you to embrace that fear, dance with it and transform it into love. Because, at the end of the day, that's what we're all looking for, isn't it? Love. Connection. Oneness.

In the next chapter, we will explore how we can channel sexual energy, which is such a potent and transformative force, into our creativity. But for now, I invite you to reflect on what we have shared today. How can you integrate tantra into your relationships? How can you create more space for presence, authentic communication and sacred sexuality in your life?

This is your journey, dear reader, and I am here with you, every step of the way. Remember, you are braver than you think, stronger than you look and more loved than you can imagine.

We are coming to the end of this chapter, but in reality, we are at the beginning of a journey, of a personal transformation and of the relationships you maintain. The tantric view of relationships that we have explored is one that honors the divinity in each of us, that celebrates the union of the feminine and masculine, and that sees every act of love as a reflection of the cosmic union of energy and consciousness.

Tantra invites us to relate to our loved ones in a more conscious, more present and more loving way. It invites us to see our partner not only as an individual with needs, desires and fears, but as a reflection of the divine. This vision has the potential to transform our relationships, to make them deeper, more authentic and more fulfilling.

The journey we have taken so far is only the beginning. There is much more to discover and experience on the path of tantra. Remember, it is a path of exploration and experimentation. There is no one "right way" to do it. What works for one, may not work for another. So I encourage you to take this journey as an opportunity to learn, grow and transform.

And speaking of transformation, in the next chapter, we will explore one of the most revolutionary teachings of tantra: the sublimation of sexual energy. We will delve into how we can channel this powerful energy into our creativity and self-realization.

You may be thinking, "Sexual energy and creativity? How are they related?" Or perhaps you are intrigued by the idea that sexual energy can be more than just a force for procreation or physical pleasure. Whatever your reaction, I encourage you to keep an open mind and come with me on this exciting journey.

So pack your bags, because the next chapter will take us into new and exciting territory. I am excited about what we will discover together. As always, I'm with you every step of the way, as we continue to walk this path together, in the ecstasy of now.

Chapter 19: Sublimated Sexual Energy: Channeling Creative Power

Have you ever felt a spark of inspiration, a current of creativity that seems to flow directly from within you to the outside world? Have you wondered where that energy comes from and how you could increase it? Could it be possible that it is somehow connected to your sexuality?

I want you to reflect for a moment. Think about the great artists, the musicians, the writers, the dancers. Think about the people you admire for their creativity and their ability to bring something beautiful and meaningful into the world. Could it be that they are somehow channeling their sexual energy in a way that allows them to create in that way?

In this chapter, we will explore the tantric idea of sublimated sexual energy and how it can be channeled to empower our creativity. You see, tantra teaches us that our sexual energy is much more than simply a force for procreation or physical pleasure. It is a potent source of life, of vitality, of inspiration.

Don't you find it fascinating? This is a concept that can totally change the way you view your own sexuality and creativity. It is a path that can lead you to discover new forms of self-expression and self-fulfillment. But, before we start walking down it, we need to understand what exactly it means to sublimate sexual energy and how this process works.

The word "sublimate" comes from the Latin "sublimare", which means "to elevate". In the context of tantra, sublimating sexual energy implies elevating it, transmuting it from its most basic and physical state to a more subtle and spiritual state. It is not about repressing or denying our sexuality, but using it as a force for our personal and spiritual evolution.

In more practical terms, sublimating sexual energy involves learning to manage it so that it does not remain trapped in our lower energy centers, but can ascend and expand throughout our body and mind. In this way, we can harness its full potential to nourish our being at all levels: physical, emotional, mental and spiritual.

Now, you are probably wondering how this is done. How can we learn to sublimate our sexual energy and use it to enhance our creativity? How can we transform this latent potential into a living, vibrant force?

These are profound questions, questions that invite us to explore the mysteries of our own energy and potential. And that is precisely what we will do in this chapter.

So I invite you to sit comfortably, take a deep breath and open yourself to the possibility of discovering something new about yourself and the incredible power within you. Because, as you will see, sublimating your sexual energy and channeling it into your creativity is a path full of surprises and revelations.

Are you ready to embark on this journey? Are you ready to discover a new aspect of your sexuality and your creative capacity? Here we go!

Let's start by taking a look at history. The idea of sublimated sexual energy is not something new. In fact, it has been present in different cultures and spiritual traditions throughout the centuries. From ancient Hindu and Taoist mystics to Renaissance philosophers and modern psychologists, many have spoken of the connection between sexuality and creativity, and how we can learn to transmute our sexual energy into creative energy.

One of the first to talk about this was Sigmund Freud, the father of psychoanalysis. In his work "Three Essays on the Theory of Sexuality" (1905), Freud proposed the idea of "sublimation" as a psychological mechanism in which sexual energies are redirected into socially acceptable activities, such as art or science. According to Freud, all great artists, scientists and leaders are people who have learned to sublimate their sexual impulses into creative energy.

Later, Carl Gustav Jung, a disciple and later critic of Freud, took this idea even further. In his studies on the psychology of creativity, Jung observed that sexual energy can be sublimated not only in art or science, but in any kind of activity that requires imagination and inspiration. In Jung's words, "the libido is the energy that fuels every creative act".

However, the idea of sublimating sexual energy is not limited to Western psychology. In the East, in traditions such as Tantra and Taoism, this concept has been an integral part of their philosophy and spiritual practice for millennia.

In tantra, sexual energy is seen as a manifestation of divine energy, a sacred power that can be used for spiritual enlightenment. By sublimating this energy, tantra practitioners seek to attain higher states of consciousness and union with the divine. And, as mentioned earlier, this energy is not only used for meditation and prayer, but also for creativity and artistic expression.

Do you realize the importance of all this? Do you realize how our perception of sexuality and creativity changes when we see that they are interconnected, that they are two sides of the same coin?

Perhaps you are now beginning to see your sexuality and your creativity with new eyes. Perhaps you are beginning to understand that, instead of repressing or ignoring your sexuality, you can learn to honor it and channel it in ways that benefit you and others.

And that, my dear reader, is precisely what I propose in this chapter. I propose that you embark on a journey of discovery and exploration. I propose that you learn to sublimate your sexual energy and use it to enhance your creativity. I propose that you discover for yourself what it means to live fully your sexuality and your creativity.

Are you ready to embark on this journey? Are you willing to explore new possibilities and open yourself to new ways of being and creating? Let's dive into this exciting topic together!

Let's talk about some practical examples of how you can begin to sublimate your sexual energy and channel it into your creativity. You can take it as a starting point, a map to begin your journey.

In his book Cultivating Male Sexual Energy (1989), Mantak Chia, a contemporary Taoist master, presents a series of exercises and meditations designed to help men learn to control and channel their sexual energy. Although the book is aimed specifically at men, many of the practices he proposes are equally applicable to women.

One of the most basic exercises that Chia proposes is conscious breathing. According to him, simply by becoming aware of our breathing and learning to breathe in a deeper and more relaxed way, we can begin to manage our sexual energy more effectively.

Imagine this: you are sitting quietly, becoming aware of each inhalation and exhalation. With each inhalation, you visualize your sexual energy rising from your lower centers to your heart and head. With each exhalation, you visualize how this energy expands throughout your body, filling you with vitality and creativity.

Another exercise that Chia proposes is meditation on the chakras. In chapter 10, we already explored the importance of the chakras in tantra and how they can help us manage our sexual energy. In the practice Chia proposes, you focus on each of your chakras, from the lowest to the highest, and visualize how your sexual energy flows and expands through them.

You can imagine it this way: you are sitting quietly, focusing your attention on your root chakra, the center of your sexual energy. You visualize how this energy begins to move up your spine, passing through each of your chakras. With each chakra it passes through, you feel your energy transform and become more subtle, lighter. When it reaches your crown chakra, at the top of your head, you feel it expand and pour through your entire being, filling you with inspiration and creativity.

Both exercises are simple, but powerful. They are a way to begin to become aware of your sexual energy and learn to manage it so that you can sublimate it and channel it into your creativity.

Now, it is important to keep in mind that these exercises are only a starting point. True sublimation of sexual energy is a long and deep path, requiring practice and dedication. But, as the ancient Chinese proverb says, "the journey of a thousand miles begins with a single step." And these exercises can be that first step.

Are you ready to take that step? Are you willing to embark on this journey of transformation and growth?

As Carl Jung mentions in "The Psychology of Transmutation" (1940), sexual energy is not only a physical force, but also a psychic one. It is an energy that can nourish our creativity and fuel our inspiration. But, in order to harness it in this way, we need to learn to handle it with awareness and respect.

The poet William Blake, in his work "The Marriage of Heaven and Hell" (1790), said that "energy is the only life and is of the body; and reason is the surrounding boundary or circumference of energy". For Blake, energy, and specifically sexual energy, was a source of life and creativity. But, in order to harness it in this way, we need to learn to manage it with awareness and respect.

What does this imply in practice? It involves learning to be present, to pay attention to our sensations and emotions. It involves learning to breathe consciously, to relax our body and mind. It involves learning to meditate, to connect with our energy centers and to visualize how our sexual energy rises and expands throughout our being.

On this path towards the sublimation of sexual energy, it is important to remember that it is not a race, but a journey. It is not about reaching a destination, but about enjoying the journey. So I invite you to take this path calmly, patiently, with love and respect for yourself. Remember, as we mentioned in chapter 7, the art of surrender is fundamental to overcome blocks and resistances on this path.

You've come a long way here, but the journey is not over yet. In the next chapter, "The Journey Continues: Personal Growth and Transformation Through Tantra," we will delve into how you can apply these practices and concepts in your daily life and how they can help you grow and evolve as an individual. It is a journey of self-discovery and self-knowledge, of learning and growth. I invite you to move forward with courage and openness, with curiosity and love for yourself.

I am excited to join you on this journey and look forward to seeing how your journey continues. Remember: you are an incredibly powerful and creative being. Your sexual energy is a formidable force that can fuel your inspiration and creativity. And, with the practices and concepts we've explored in this chapter, you have the tools to begin to unleash that potential.

Are you ready to move forward? Are you ready to discover the power and beauty of your sublimated sexual energy? See you in the next chapter. Until then, keep exploring, keep learning, keep growing. see you soon!

Chapter 20: The Journey Continues: Personal Growth and Transformation Through Tantra

So here we are, dear reader. Did you realize that you have already come a long way from the beginning? We have shared moments of learning, laughter, wonder and doubt, but most importantly, we have grown together. And, although this chapter may have the number 20 engraved on its cover, I want you to know that this is not the end. As the title says, the journey continues.

Let me ask you a question: Have you ever felt that feeling of stagnation, that your life has reached a dead end? It's that feeling of being in a labyrinth and not finding the exit, of repeating over and over again the same patterns, as if you were trapped in an infinite loop. I'm sure it rings a bell, doesn't it? We've all been there at some point.

Sometimes life can seem like a frustrating board game, where every time we think we are about to reach the finish line, something takes us back to square one. It's as if we have a preordained destiny and every attempt to change it only takes us back to the same starting point. But what if I told you that this is not the case? What if I told you that you have the ability to change your life, to transform yourself, to grow and evolve in ways you can't even imagine?

This is exactly what Tantra proposes to us. As we have already mentioned in previous chapters (especially in chapters 6 and 19), Tantra is a path of self-knowledge and self-development. It is a practice that allows us to explore our body and mind, our sexuality and spirituality, our individual being and our connection with the whole. But Tantra is not only a series of techniques and practices; it is also a philosophy of life, a way of understanding and experiencing the world.

That is why, in this chapter, we intend to delve deeper into the topic of personal growth and transformation through Tantra. We will explore how Tantra can help you overcome blocks and resistances, release old patterns and limiting beliefs, unleash your potential and become the best version of yourself.

I am convinced that this chapter will be of great use to you, whether you have already started your tantric path or you are thinking of taking the first steps. Because Tantra is a journey, and as in every journey, there is always something new to discover, there is always a new perspective to explore, there is always a new horizon to conquer.

So, are you ready to continue the journey? Are you ready to embark on this adventure of growth and transformation? I assure you it will be an exciting journey, full of discoveries and surprises. And remember, no matter how far you go, there will always be a new horizon to explore, there will always be something more to learn, there will always be a new adventure to live. Because, as an ancient tantric proverb says, "the path is the destination".

Okay, dear reader, let's get down to business. First, let's see how the practice of Tantra can help you free yourself from old patterns and limiting beliefs. We all have, to a greater or lesser extent, beliefs and patterns that limit us. Some of these beliefs were instilled in us in our childhood, others we acquired throughout our lives, and many times we are not even aware that they exist.

Have you ever felt that you always end up in the same situation, as if you were trapped in a vicious circle? This is what Carl Jung, the famous Swiss psychologist, called "the shadow". According to Jung, the shadow is the part of ourselves that we reject or deny, and therefore remains hidden in our subconscious. But even if we ignore it, the shadow continues to influence our lives, generating repetitive and self-destructive patterns of behavior.

But don't worry, Tantra has a solution for this. The practice of Tantra invites us to explore our shadow, to recognize and accept all parts of ourselves, even those we find uncomfortable or painful. In this way, we can free ourselves from old patterns and beliefs that limit us and begin to live a more authentic and fulfilling life.

And this is where the tantric techniques we have been learning throughout this book come into play. Remember, for example, the tantric meditation we explored in Chapter 11, or the tantric massage in Chapter 15. These techniques not only help us release physical and emotional tension, but also allow us to explore and transform our limiting beliefs and patterns.

On the other hand, Tantra also provides us with tools to unleash our potential and become the best version of ourselves. As the philosopher and psychologist Abraham Maslow said, "what one can be, one must be". Maslow, known for his theory of self-actualization, argued that we all have an inherent potential that seeks expression and fulfillment. And Tantra shares this vision.

Indeed, we could say that self-realization is the ultimate goal of Tantra. As we mentioned in chapter 7, Tantra teaches us to surrender ourselves completely, to live each moment with total intensity and authenticity. And this surrender, this authenticity, is what allows us to unleash our potential and become the best version of ourselves.

Now, what exactly does it mean to "be the best version of yourself"? Well, this may vary from person to person, as each of us is unique and has our own path to follow. But, in general terms, we could say that being the best version of oneself means living according to our values and principles, following our dreams and passions, developing our skills and talents, and contributing to the well-being of others and the planet. And, of course, it also means enjoying life, experiencing pleasure and joy, and celebrating our existence in this wonderful universe.

To better understand how Tantra can help us become the best version of ourselves, let us take a look at a story told by tantric master Osho in his book "Tantra: The Supreme Understanding" (1975). In this story, a young prince, desperate to find his life's purpose, abandons his kingdom and retreats to the jungle to meditate. After many years of meditation, the prince attains enlightenment and returns to his kingdom. But instead of returning to his former life of luxury and pleasure, he decides to devote himself to serving his people and teaching them what he has learned. And despite the difficulties and challenges, the prince feels happier and more satisfied than ever.

What is the message of this story? That self-realization, being the best version of ourselves, is not a matter of ego or vanity, but of authenticity and service. It is, as the poet Kahlil Gibran said, "giving the best you have" and "knowing that what you give is truly yours".

And now, dear reader, let me share with you an example closer to our times. Imagine a successful executive, with a high salary, a luxury car and a nice house. But this executive is not happy. He feels empty and unfulfilled, and realizes that his life has no meaning. Then, one day, he discovers Tantra and decides to try it. At first, he feels a little uncomfortable and insecure, but little by little he begins to notice changes in his life. He begins to feel more alive, more present, more connected to his body and emotions. He begins to free himself from his fears and blocks, to explore new forms of pleasure and relationships. And, most importantly, he begins to discover who he really is and what he wants from life.

This executive could be any one of us. It could be us who, like him, feel dissatisfied with our lives and are looking for something more. And, like him, we can find in Tantra a path to authenticity, fulfillment and happiness.

Of course, this does not mean that Tantra is an easy path. As in any journey, there will be moments of doubt and confusion, moments of pain and difficulty. But, as the poet Robert Frost said, "the only way out is through." And, though the road may be difficult, the destination is well worth it.

So, dear reader, I invite you to keep moving forward, to keep exploring, to keep growing and transforming yourself. I invite you to keep being curious, to keep being brave, to keep being yourself. Because you are the key, you are the way, you are the path, you are the treasure. The transformation you seek is not in some distant place or in some esoteric teaching, but in yourself, in your own experience, in your own wisdom. As the Sufi poet and philosopher Rumi said, "the light you seek is in your own courtyard".

I hope these concepts and examples have helped you to understand and appreciate the importance of personal growth and transformation on the path of Tantra. As we have seen, Tantra is not only a sexual or spiritual practice, but also a path of self-discovery and self-realization. A path that leads us to know and accept our true nature, to unleash our potential and to live a more authentic, fulfilling and satisfying life.

Dear reader, you have done an incredible job in getting this far, in immersing yourself in these pages and opening yourself to new perspectives and possibilities. I congratulate you on your courage, your curiosity and your commitment to your own growth and well-being. You are, without a doubt, a true adventurer of the spirit, a true seeker of ecstasy.

But this is not the end of the road. In fact, it is only the beginning. The journey of Tantra is a never-ending journey, a journey of constant learning, exploration and evolution. And, like all good journeys, it is a journey that is most enjoyable when it is shared.

Therefore, I invite you to keep moving forward, to keep exploring, to keep growing and transforming yourself. And, above all, I invite you to share your journey, your experiences and your discoveries with others. Because, as the great Carl Sagan said, "we are the way the cosmos knows itself".

And now, dear reader, prepare your spirit for the next chapter of our journey, Chapter 21: "Modern Tantrics: Women and the Power of Sexual Energy". In it, you will discover how women are reinventing Tantra and using their sexual power and energy to heal, empower and transform the world. I promise it will be an exciting, inspiring and deeply liberating journey. So, are you ready to continue exploring the fascinating world of Tantra? Here we go!

Chapter 21: Modern Tantrics: Women and the Power of Sexual Energy

Have you ever noticed, dear reader, that sparkle in the eyes of a woman who feels self-confident, who lives her sexual energy to the fullest and emanates a magnetic force? Hasn't it made you feel a mixture of fascination, respect and longing? If the answer is yes, then you are in the presence of a Modern Tantric.

But what does it mean to be a Modern Tantric? And more importantly, what does it have to do with sexual energy and Tantra? Allow me to illuminate this path of transformation and empowerment. If you are ready to embark on this journey of self-knowledge and liberation, I promise that your perspective on the power and potential of feminine sexual energy will radically change.

Modern Tantricas are women who have unlocked and channeled their sexual energy, not only to enhance their pleasure and intimacy, but also to transform all facets of their lives. They are women who have learned to use their sexual energy as a source of power, creativity, healing and connection to the divine.

Why is it important to talk about Modern Tantrics and the power of female sexual energy? Because, dear reader, for too long, women's sexuality has been repressed, stigmatized, feared and misunderstood. But Tantra offers us a different perspective, a vision that honors and celebrates female sexuality as a source of life, beauty, wisdom and power.

This path is not for every woman. It requires courage, patience, openness and honesty with oneself. It requires challenging social norms, dismantling limiting beliefs and overcoming fears and insecurities. But I assure you, dear reader, the rewards are immense.

And I want to make it clear: being a Modern Tantric has nothing to do with how many orgasms you can have, what positions you can do in bed, or how many lovers you have had. Being a Modern Tantric has to do with how you relate to yourself, your body, your sexual energy and the world around you.

So what does this concept of Modern Tantric mean to you, dear reader? How does this vision of feminine sexuality resonate with you? What possibilities does it open up for you, whether you are a man or a woman? I invite you to reflect on these questions and to open yourself to new ways of thinking and living your sexuality. Because, as the great feminist and philosopher Simone de Beauvoir said in "The Second Sex" (1949), "sexuality is the struggle of life against death".

And now, dear reader, let us enter the fascinating world of Modern Tantric and discover how, through Tantra, women can release and channel their sexual energy to transform their lives and their world.

Have you ever wondered, dear reader, what it really means to release and channel sexual energy? It's not about uninhibited surrender to carnal pleasures, although that may be part of the process. It is something much deeper and more transcendental. Sexual energy is a vital energy, it is the energy of creation and life itself. And when a woman connects with that energy and learns to manage it, she becomes a force of nature.

Margot Anand, in her book "The Art of Sexual Ecstasy: The Tantric Path to Sexual Health and Fulfillment" (1996), talks about how sexual energy can be a gateway to higher states of consciousness and experiences of ecstasy. Can you imagine, dear reader, what it would be like if every act of love and pleasure became a meditation, a sacred ritual of union with the cosmos?

But it is not just about great mystical experiences. Sexual energy also has very practical and tangible applications in a woman's daily life. For example, it can help increase self-esteem and self-confidence, improve health and physical well-being, awaken creativity and deepen relationships.

Remember, dear reader, when we talked in chapter 19 about sublimated sexual energy and how it can be channeled into creativity and productivity? Well, this is exactly what Modern Tantrics do. They use their sexual energy, not only for pleasure and intimacy, but also to fuel their work, their projects, their art and their activism.

These women are true revolutionaries. They challenge society's norms and expectations and blaze new trails of authenticity and empowerment. Their courage and passion are truly inspiring.

Yes, it may sound far away, very different from your reality. But I want you to know, my reader friend, that all women have the potential to become Modern Tantric. It doesn't matter the age, sexual orientation, experience or circumstances. All it takes is the willingness to explore and learn, the courage to challenge old beliefs and patterns, and the commitment to one's own growth and transformation.

So, dear reader, are you willing to explore this new vision of female sexuality? Are you willing to challenge your own beliefs and expectations? Are you willing to open yourself to new ways of experiencing and understanding pleasure, love and intimacy?

If the answer is yes, then welcome to this exciting journey of discovery and transformation. I promise you that it will be an adventure full of surprises, challenges, learning and, above all, a lot of pleasure and joy. Because, as the great writer Anais Nin said, "Life shrinks or expands in proportion to our courage". And you, dear reader, are about to expand your life in ways you never imagined.

Let me now share with you some concrete examples of how Modern Tantric Women have used their sexual energy to transform their lives and their world. As you listen to these stories, I invite you to ask yourself, how could I apply this in my own life? How could I, whether I am a woman or a man, learn to release and channel my sexual energy in such powerful and creative ways?

Consider the case of Sophia, a woman who had always felt a big block in her sexuality. After years of struggling with feelings of shame and guilt, she decided to enter the world of Tantra. During her journey, Sophia faced her fears and traumas, learned to love and accept her body as it is, and began to experience her sexuality in ways she had never imagined. Now, Sophia is a Modern Tantric, a woman who radiates powerful sexual energy and uses this energy to empower other women through her work as a coach and therapist.

Or think of Anaya, an artist who had always had difficulty finding the inspiration and motivation to create. When she discovered Tantra and began to connect with her sexual energy, her creativity overflowed. Now, Anaya creates stunning and vibrant artwork that reflects her journey of self-exploration and sexual liberation. Her sexual energy has become the muse that fuels her art.

These are just two examples of how Modern Tantrics are transforming their lives and their world. But there are many more stories to be discovered. And perhaps, dear reader, your own story is waiting to be written.

Make no mistake, the path of Modern Tantric is not an easy one. As Regina Thomashauer points out in her book "Pussy: A Reclamation" (2016), this journey requires facing the shadow, fears, taboos and traumas. But it is also a path of liberation, empowerment and profound transformation.

Tantra teaches us that every woman is a divine being, an embodiment of the Goddess, and that her sexuality is an expression of this divine. When a woman connects with this truth and learns to release and channel her sexual energy, she becomes a Modern Tantric.

So, dear reader, what do you think of this vision of Modern Tantric? How does this new way of understanding and living female sexuality resonate with you? I invite you to reflect on these questions and open yourself to new ways of thinking and experiencing your sexuality.

Are you ready to continue this journey? Are you ready to discover more about the power of sexual energy and how it can transform your life and your world? If the answer is yes, then grab my hand and let's continue together. I'm here with you, supporting you every step of this exciting journey. And remember, as the brilliant author Clarissa Pinkola Estés said in "Women Who Run with the Wolves" (1992), "Strong women are those who have made their lives a sacred journey."

In exploring the fascinating world of Modern Tantric, we have embarked together on a journey of self-discovery and transformation. We have seen how sexual energy, when released and channeled in a conscious and loving way, can become a powerful force for change and creativity. Through Sophia and Anaya's stories, we have glimpsed the potential that is awakened when a woman steps onto the path of Tantra.

Some of the ideas presented in this chapter may have challenged or even puzzled you. You may wonder how you might apply these teachings in your own life. Let me remind you, dear reader, that Tantra is a path of self-exploration and self-discovery. There is no "right" way to do it. Your journey will be unique and personal, and will take you exactly where you need to be.

Before ending this chapter, I want to remind you once again of the importance of your relationship with yourself. As I mentioned in Chapter 7, "The Art of Surrender," the first and most important step in any journey of self-discovery is learning to love and accept yourself as you are.

Dear reader, in this chapter we have explored together the powerful force of Modern Tantric and its conscious and loving use of sexual energy. But this is only the beginning. There is much more to discover in the wonderful world of Tantra.

In the next chapter, "Male Awakening: Masculinity and Sensitivity in Tantra," we will focus on male awakening. If you have marveled at the power of Modern Tantric, wait until you see how men are also awakening and honoring their own sexual energy. We will see how sensitivity and strength can coexist in the essence of a man, and how Tantra can offer a new model of masculinity, away from limiting stereotypes. If you identify as a man, you will find here valuable tools to rediscover your authentic essence and unleash your potential. And if you identify as a woman, you will be able to better understand how to accompany men in this awakening process.

So, are you ready to keep exploring, are you ready to open yourself to new ways of seeing, feeling and experiencing your sexuality and your being? I invite you to continue this journey, and remember, I am always here, by your side, to accompany and support you every step of the way.

See you in the next chapter, dear reader. Until then, I wish you love, light and blessings on your way.

Chapter 22: Awakening the Man: Masculinity and Sensitivity in Tantra

What does it mean to be a man in today's world, and how does masculinity relate to Tantra? Dear reader, in this chapter we will delve into these sometimes uncharted and challenging terrains, hoping to shed some light on what it really means to be a man in the modern age and how Tantra can help define a new masculinity, one that honors both strength and sensitivity.

Masculinity, like femininity, has been subject to numerous stereotypes and social expectations for centuries. But what is the truth behind these preconceived ideas, and what role do they play in shaping our identity and self-concept? These are important questions we should all be asking ourselves, regardless of how we identify ourselves.

The answer to these questions can be complex and multifaceted, but at the same time it can be surprisingly simple: being a man, at its core, is not so much about what you do or how you behave, but about how you feel about yourself and how you relate to the world around you.

In today's society, men are often taught to be strong, to be brave, to be providers. They are encouraged to suppress their emotions, to resist showing vulnerability. In the world of Tantra, however, these notions are being challenged and revised. In Tantra, both strength and vulnerability are celebrated, both action and receptivity are honored.

Tantric masculinity, therefore, is not a negation of traditional masculinity, but rather an expansion of it. It is a recognition that there is much more to being a man than society often suggests. It is a path to greater authenticity, greater connection with self and others, and ultimately greater fulfillment and satisfaction in life.

Now, what does all this mean in practical terms? How does tantric masculinity manifest in everyday life? And, more importantly, how can you begin to cultivate it in yourself? Throughout this chapter, we will explore these questions in depth. But before we do, I would like to invite you to pause and reflect on what masculinity means to you.

How has your idea of masculinity influenced you in your life? In what ways has it served you, and in what areas may it have limited your personal growth and development? Remember, there are no right or wrong answers here. There is only your truth, your experience. And it is through this honest and authentic self-inquiry that true awakening can happen. So, are you ready to step into this journey of self-discovery and transformation? Let's get to it.

Now, you are not alone in this exploration of masculinity. Many have navigated these waters before us, and their words and insights can offer valuable guidance. One of these is renowned psychologist and author Robert Moore, who in his influential work "King, Warrior, Magician, Lover: Rediscovering the Archetypes of the Mature Masculine" (1990), speaks of the need for a renewal of the masculine image and proposes a deeper look at male archetypes.

Moore argues that, beyond stereotypes and societal expectations, there are four primary archetypes of masculinity: the king, the warrior, the magician and the lover. Each of these archetypes represents an essential aspect of masculinity and together they form an integrated and balanced model of what it means to be a man.

But what do these archetypes have to do with Tantra? A lot, actually. Remember chapter 8, where we talked about polarity and explored the masculine and feminine energies? Well, Moore's archetypes can help us to better understand the different manifestations of masculine energy and to cultivate a more balanced and harmonious relationship with it.

For example, the king archetype speaks of the ability to lead and take responsibility, but also of the importance of generosity and service to others. And what better form of service than honoring and respecting your partner's body and energy during a tantric practice?

Or consider the archetype of the lover, which represents the ability to connect emotionally and enjoy sensory pleasure. These qualities are fundamental in Tantra, where emotional connection and exploration of pleasure are key elements.

So how can you cultivate these archetypes in yourself? Well, this is where Tantra really shines. Through its meditation, breathing and massage practices, Tantra offers you powerful tools to connect with these aspects of yourself and bring them into the light.

But remember, this is not a quick or easy transformation path. It requires patience, perseverance and, above all, authenticity.

As poet and philosopher Ralph Waldo Emerson wrote in his essay "Self-Reliance" (1841), "To be what we are and become what we are capable of being is the only purpose of life." So, my friend, I encourage you to embark on this journey with courage and authenticity. There is nothing more courageous than being yourself. And on the path of Tantra, there is nothing more sacred than that.

Let us then continue to delve deeper into this fascinating and sometimes challenging path of male awakening in Tantra, illustrating with concrete examples for you to practice in your mind. A good example of this can be the tantric practice of conscious breathing.

Imagine a man who throughout his life has been trained to show strength, to show no emotions, to compete, to win. This man may feel that his body is something to be controlled, dominated. He may even have disconnected from his body to such a degree that it is difficult for him to identify his own needs and desires. This man, when he approaches Tantra, may encounter strong internal resistances, he may feel that his concept of masculinity is challenged.

Then, one day, he decides to participate in a Tantra workshop. At first, he is uncomfortable, out of his comfort zone. But little by little, as he practices conscious breathing, he begins to notice a change. He feels his body relax, the tensions melt away. And then, something extraordinary happens: you begin to feel.

Feel the delicacy of the fabric of your clothes against your skin, the warmth of your own breathing, the rhythmic pulse of your heart. She discovers sensations she has never experienced before. She realizes that her body is not an adversary to be controlled, but an ally, a temple of sensations, a portal to a new way of being.

This man is an example of how Tantra can transform our relationship with our own masculinity. Through simple but powerful practices such as conscious breathing, we can learn to listen to our body, honor it and care for it. We can learn to feel, connect and celebrate our masculinity in a way that is nurturing and enriching.

Another example is meditation, another central tool in Tantra. Think of a man who has always felt disconnected from his emotions. Through meditation, he can learn to observe his emotions without judging them, to welcome them and allow them to exist. He can discover that it is possible to be a man and cry, to feel fear, to express love. He can learn that true strength is not found in repression, but in acceptance and vulnerability.

So, my friend, Tantra offers a path of awakening for the modern man, a path that invites you to explore, discover and embrace all facets of your masculinity. A path that invites you to truly be yourself.

Do you notice how little by little the old-fashioned idea that masculinity is synonymous with hardness and dominance is fading away? Do you perceive how the tantric path leads us to an awakening where masculinity and sensitivity can go hand in hand, without implying a contradiction?

It is as if we were stripping away a flower, layer by layer, revealing the purest essence of what it means to be human in a context of full consciousness. As if we were erasing ancient inscriptions in stone, only to rewrite a new script, one that allows men to be fully human, to feel deeply, to love intensely and to live authentically.

This awakening is not an easy path, I admit. You will need courage to look inside yourself, patience to unlearn and relearn, and an open heart to accept all facets of your being. But, my friend, I can assure you that the journey is worth it. You will not only transform your relationship with yourself, but also your relationships with others. You will become a beacon of love, acceptance and understanding, lighting the way for other men who are also seeking an awakening.

And with this, we conclude our journey through Chapter 22, "Awakening the Man: Masculinity and Sensitivity in Tantra." Throughout this journey, we have explored how Tantra can help men shed the old bonds of traditional masculinity and embark on a path of self-discovery and authenticity.

I thank you for joining me on this journey and hope that what we have explored together will help you on your personal path of growth and transformation. Ready to move forward? I invite you to join me in the next chapter! There we will dive into the interesting world of Tantric Massage and Culture, where we will challenge some established norms and beliefs. I promise, it will be a fascinating journey full of surprises and discoveries. See you there? Until then, keep the flame of your heart alive!

Chapter 23: Tantric Massage and Culture: Challenging Norms and Beliefs

Join me on this fascinating journey, dive into the little explored waters of the intersection between Tantric Massage and culture. This is not a journey for the faint of heart, it is a challenge, a questioning of the normativity and beliefs we have inherited and adopted. But don't worry, I promise to keep you afloat, to guide you with the light of Tantric wisdom as we dismantle together preconceived notions about sexuality and pleasure.

Have you ever wondered how cultural beliefs and norms have influenced your sex life? How they have shaped your expectations, your desires, your sense of what is right or wrong? Have you ever stopped to think about how much of what you believe and feel is really yours and how much has been imposed on you by the culture you grew up in?

Culture is an intricate canvas woven with threads of history, politics, economics, and each of these dimensions has something to say about sexuality and pleasure. Some cultures worship the body and celebrate sexuality, such as the ancient civilization of India, where Tantra was born. Others may see the body and sexual pleasure as sinful or impure, creating a strong division between the spiritual and the physical.

However, it is important to remember that culture is not a monolithic block. There are a variety of beliefs and practices within each culture, and each individual has the ability to question, reinterpret and change cultural norms. This is where Tantric Massage comes into play, as a powerful tool to challenge restrictive cultural norms and cultivate a healthier and more satisfying relationship with our sexuality.

Are you ready for this adventure, for this courageous exploration of the intersections between Tantric Massage and culture? I assure you that it will not only change the way you view your sexuality, but it will also transform your relationship with your body, with your partner and with yourself. So, take a deep breath, open your mind and heart, and join me on this journey into the unknown.

We have already opened the door, and now we will delve even deeper into this fascinating cultural labyrinth. Let's start with a look back at the history of Tantra and how it has evolved in different cultures. Did you know that Tantric Massage, as we know it today, is the result of thousands of years of practice and experimentation?

Yes, you may be surprised to learn that Tantra has its roots in ancient India, and has been influenced and shaped by a variety of cultures and religious traditions over the centuries. Despite being marginalized and suppressed by colonial forces and restrictive cultural norms, Tantra has survived, mutated and adapted. Even in the face of adversity, the seed of Tantra never stopped growing.

Like the river that flows ceaselessly and changes the landscape, Tantra has influenced and changed the cultures it has touched. Through Tantric Massage, we have seen how norms and beliefs about sexuality and pleasure can be questioned, challenged, and ultimately transformed.

In this regard, a book published in 1989 by cultural anthropologist William Jankowiak entitled "Sex, Death, and Hierarchy in a Chinese City" comes to mind. Jankowiak explored how cultural changes in China have affected sexuality and intimate relationships. She found that ideas about sexuality were strongly influenced by politics, economics, and reliGu Script.

In particular, Jankowiak discussed how Tantric Massage challenged social and sexual norms in contemporary China, providing a safe space for people to explore their sexuality and pleasure in ways that the dominant culture often repressed or denied. This study is just one of many that reveal how Tantric Massage can act as a counterculture, challenging restrictive norms and beliefs.

Now, I want you to take a moment to reflect on this. Can you see how your culture has influenced your own sexuality? How it has shaped your desires, your fears, your expectations? And most importantly, can you see how Tantric Massage can be a way to challenge and transform those norms and beliefs?

Now, let me tell you a story that clearly illustrates the clash and eventual blending of cultures. At the heart of this story is Tantric Massage, playing a crucial role in the intersection of two worlds.

Imagine a small village in Thailand, a hidden gem where tradition is still going strong. Here, traditional Thai massage, also known as "Nuad Boran", has been passed down from generation to generation. But one day, a foreign traveler arrives in the village. He has been exploring the world, learning about various massage techniques, and on his journey, he came across tantric massage.

That traveler decides to share his knowledge with the townspeople. At first, there is resistance. Tantric Massage is different, it is unknown. Some even see it as a threat to their traditional form of massage. But little by little, people become curious. They try the technique, experience the tantric energy, and begin to appreciate it.

Then, the fusion begins. The elements of Tantric Massage begin to integrate with Nuad Boran. The result is something new, something vibrant. It is a form of massage that carries the energy of both cultures, challenging and at the same time enriching their established beliefs and practices.

This story, dear reader, is but one example. It has happened and continues to happen in countless ways and in countless places. But always at the heart of this clash and eventual blending of cultures, we find Tantric Massage, defying norms, breaking down barriers, creating bridges.

Here, author and psychologist David Deida, in his book "The Way of the Superior Man" (1997), gives us a relevant insight. Deida argues that each individual and each culture has its own ways of expressing and experiencing sexuality. But he also suggests that all cultures can benefit from openness to new forms of sexual and sensual expression, such as Tantra.

Imagine, for a moment, what it would be like if the practice of Tantric Massage became more widespread in your own culture. How would attitudes towards sexuality change? How would relationships transform? How would you transform yourself? Can you see the power of Tantric Massage to challenge norms and beliefs?

Now, sit with me here, in this imaginary space where culture and beliefs meet and merge, and reflect on what we have discovered together in this chapter.

We have talked about the power of Tantric Massage to challenge cultural norms and beliefs. We have discussed how the practice of Tantra can open new doors of perception, encouraging people to explore and accept freer and more conscious forms of sexuality. And we have seen how, in doing so, Tantric Massage can act as an agent of personal, but also social and cultural change and growth.

Because, if you think about it, every time you challenge your own beliefs, every time you open yourself up to new ideas and practices, you are changing not only yourself, but also the world around you. You are becoming a catalyst for broader change. As French sociologist and philosopher Michel Foucault wrote in The History of Sexuality (1976), "Where there is power, there is resistance."

And isn't this resistance a sign of growth, of evolution, of transformation? Isn't this resistance the seed of the personal and cultural revolution that Tantric Massage can unleash?

Look at it this way: every time you choose to explore the path of Tantra, every time you practice Tantric Massage, you are not only nurturing your own growth and transformation. You are also, in one way or another, challenging cultural norms and beliefs, you are pushing the boundaries of what is considered possible and acceptable, and you are contributing to a deeper and broader change in society.

So I invite you, my friend, to keep exploring, keep challenging, keep growing. Because, ultimately, that is the true power and the true beauty of Tantric Massage.

And now, as we approach the end of this chapter, let me give you a preview of what's to come in the next one. We will be entering exciting and revolutionary territory: the idea of achieving enlightenment through pleasure. It's a prospect that, I'm sure, will fill you with anticipation and curiosity. So, are you ready to continue this journey with me? I hope you are. Because, after all, we're in this together.

Chapter 24: Achieving Enlightenment Through Pleasure: A Revolutionary Path

Dear reader, I invite you to sit comfortably, take a deep breath and prepare yourself for a revolutionary journey towards enlightenment. This is not a path of sacrifice and deprivation, but a path that accepts and celebrates pleasure as an intrinsic part of our existence. Don't you find it fascinating and liberating?

You have probably heard of enlightenment as a state of heightened consciousness, a spiritual awakening that is usually associated with the renunciation of the material world and sensual pleasures. However, what if I told you that there is a school of thought that, instead of rejecting pleasure, celebrates it and considers it a vehicle to enlightenment?

This is the premise of Tantra. While many spiritual traditions have adopted a negative view of the body and pleasure, labeling them distractions or temptations on the path to enlightenment, Tantra, by contrast, embraces the totality of human experience, including pleasure, as an expression of divinity. As I explained in Chapter 6: "Kundalini Awakens: Sexual Energy and Spirituality," Tantric philosophy considers sexual energy to be a form of spiritual energy, and by consciously channeling it, we can reach a higher state of consciousness.

But what does "enlightenment" really mean? And how is it possible to achieve enlightenment through pleasure?

Enlightenment is a term that has been used and redefined by various traditions and schools of thought throughout history. Although there is no single universally accepted definition, it generally refers to a state of consciousness in which we overcome the dualistic perception of ourselves and the world, achieving a profound understanding of the unity of all things. In this state, we are said to experience profound peace and freedom from suffering.

Now, when we speak of attaining enlightenment through pleasure in the context of Tantra, we are referring to the act of witnessing and consciously experiencing pleasure as a form of meditation. Through this practice, we can learn to transcend dualistic thinking and recognize the divinity in all experiences, including sensual and erotic ones.

This concept may seem somewhat revolutionary, and you may be asking yourself: how is it possible that pleasure can lead to enlightenment? I invite you to stay with me, my friend, as we explore this fascinating path together. In the following sections, we will dive into this idea, cite relevant works and authors, and offer concrete examples to help you understand and perhaps experience for yourself this revolutionary path to enlightenment through pleasure.

I hope you feel comfortable, because now, together, we are going to enter a vast ocean of wisdom and insights, surfing the waves of the words of some great thinkers and sages who have walked this path before us.

The teaching of Tantra as a path to enlightenment is not new, in fact, it has been developing over the centuries. The tantric master Osho, in his work "Tantra: The Supreme

Understanding" (1975), provided a fresh and liberating vision of Tantra, presenting it not as a technique, but as an attitude towards life. Osho encourages us to accept and celebrate all our experiences, including pleasure, as an integral part of our spiritual path. "Life is a flowing with the river of the cosmos," he said. "Flowing with it is Tantra; resisting it is samsara (suffering)."

And this flow, dear reader, is also a flow with pleasure, with joy and with ecstasy. According to Osho, when we allow ourselves to feel fully, when we are authentic to our experiences, and when we stop holding back, we are on the path to enlightenment.

This thought is also reflected in the words of Daniel Odier, another contemporary tantric master. In his book Desire: The Tantric Path to Awakening (2001), Odier explores the idea that desires and sensations are not obstacles to enlightenment, but can be used as a path to it. "Tantra invites us to embrace our sensations because they are extremely rich in wisdom," Odier tells us. Can you feel the revolution this idea brings, the liberating power it holds?

What about Tantra in the Hindu tradition? According to David Gordon White in his work Kiss of the Yogini (2003), Tantric practices in ancient India often included rituals that challenged social and religious norms, including the enjoyment of sensual pleasures. Rather than seeing these acts as sinful or distracting, they were seen as means to attain enlightenment.

As you reflect on these ideas, I want you to think about how you tend to live your own life. Are you trying to repress or ignore your desires and pleasures? Or are you willing to embrace and experience them fully, to explore them as a path to a deeper understanding of yourself and the universe? What would your life be like if you chose to embrace and celebrate your pleasures rather than fear or resist them?

Remember, I am not suggesting that you abdicate responsibility or engage in self-destructive behavior in the name of pleasure. What I am inviting you to consider is the possibility of seeing and living your pleasures in a mindful and meditative way, of learning to savor them fully, and of exploring what they can teach you about yourself and life.

So how do we apply all this to our own experience? How can we turn theory into practice? Let's look at it through a couple of concrete examples.

Imagine you are in the middle of a tantric massage. You are aware of every sensation that runs through your body, every touch, every pressure. You are in a state of deep relaxation, but also of intense awareness. Then, you feel a surge of pleasure that runs through you from the tips of your toes to the crown of your head. Instead of trying to control it, resist it or feel guilty about it, you simply observe it. You let it flow through you. You welcome it, accept it and experience it in all its depth and intensity. That surge of pleasure then becomes a vehicle for self-knowledge. What does it tell you about yourself, about your desires, about your blocks, about your capacity for joy and connection? By allowing yourself to fully experience that pleasure, you are practicing the tantric teaching that enlightenment can be achieved through pleasure.

Or maybe you are in the middle of a meditation session. You find yourself sitting quietly, observing your thoughts without judgment. Suddenly, you realize that you have a strong desire to eat a piece of chocolate cake waiting for you in the kitchen. Instead of seeing this desire as a distraction, you accept it and observe it. What emotions are associated with that desire: anxiety, anticipation, excitement, guilt? And what does this teach you about your relationship to food, to pleasure, to reward and gratification? By allowing yourself to feel and explore that desire, rather than repressing or ignoring it, you are practicing the tantric teaching that our desires can be a path to enlightenment.

But here comes a note of humor: it is very likely that, at the end of your meditation, you will find yourself running to the kitchen in search of that piece of cake. And that's perfectly fine! It's not about repressing our pleasures and desires, but learning to embrace them and live them in a more conscious and fulfilling way. If we decide to enjoy that cake, can we do so in a way that allows us to savor it fully, rather than eating it in a hurry while thinking about the next thing we have to do?

And now, I want you to think about your own experiences. Is there a situation where you have experienced pleasure or desire in a similar way? Or maybe there is a situation in your life where you could begin to apply these tantric teachings? Let me remind you that you don't need to be an expert in Tantra or have previous experience to begin to explore these ideas in your daily life. You just need an open mind, an attitude of curiosity and a willingness to experiment and learn.

Having said all this, it is important to emphasize that, although the idea of attaining enlightenment through pleasure may seem revolutionary, it is by no means new. In fact, it is a teaching that has been present in tantric traditions for thousands of years, and has been confirmed and reaffirmed by numerous authors and experts throughout history.

For example, Margot Anand, author of the book "The Art of Sexual Ecstasy" (1997), tells us how Tantra teaches us to live a life of "everyday ecstasy", in which every sensation, every emotion and every experience can become a door to enlightenment. Similarly, Daniel Odier, in his book "Desire: Tantrism and the Vital Energy of Sex" (2001), invites us to see desire as a sacred path of self-discovery and transcendence.

However, reaching this enlightenment through pleasure is not an automatic or instantaneous process. It is not enough to desire it or to read about it. It requires practice, commitment, patience and, above all, courage. Courage to face our own desires, pleasures, fears and resistances. Courage to step into the unknown, to explore new ways of being and feeling. And courage to allow ourselves to live fully, without reserve, without guilt and without fear.

If you've made it this far, you've probably already experienced some glimpses of that enlightenment through pleasure. Perhaps in a tantric massage, in a meditation, in a loving encounter, in the tasting of an exquisite meal or in the simple contemplation of a sunset. And you may ask yourself: how can I deepen this experience? How can I bring this teaching to all aspects of my life?

If you are asking yourself these questions, you are on the right track. And, dear reader, the next chapter is dedicated to just that. In it, we will explore how you can take these teachings from theory to practice, how you can move from simple intellectual understanding to true living and experience. We are going to talk about how you can integrate Tantra into your daily life, how you can become a tantric master or teacher in your own right.

Because, in the end, that is what really matters. It is not just a matter of knowing Tantra, but of living it, of making it our own, of integrating it into every aspect of our existence. And it is there, at the crossroads between knowledge and experience, where we find the true potential of Tantra.

So, I invite you to join me on this exciting journey. Together, we will explore the secrets of Tantra, learn how to live a life of fulfillment and pleasure, and discover how to achieve enlightenment through joy. Are you up for the challenge? Are you ready to embark on this journey towards your own awakening?

Chapter 25: From Practice to Mastery: Your Path to Tantric Enlightenment".

This chapter, dear reader, is an invitation. An invitation to embark on a journey, an expedition to the highest peak of your being, your true self. Are you ready to accept this challenge? Are you willing to make the necessary commitment to transcend from mere practice to true tantric mastery?

The path to tantric enlightenment is not a walk in the park. It demands from you deep commitment, perseverance, dedication and an openness of heart and mind to experiences that may challenge your preconceived ideas and take you out of your comfort zone. Are you ready to face all this?

However, do not be intimidated by this proposition, for the rewards are unparalleled. Tantric enlightenment, that state of heightened awareness and oneness with the whole, is beyond words. It cannot be described, it can only be experienced. And yes, it is possible to attain it. It is not just for monks in remote monasteries or mountaintop gurus, it is for you, here and now.

But first, what does it really mean to move from practice to mastery in the context of Tantra? What does this look like in action? And how can you, yourself, begin to walk this path?

Let us first look at the practice. As we have discussed in the previous chapters, Tantra involves a series of practices and techniques that help us connect with, expand, and sublimate our sexual energy. These include tantric massage, meditation, pranayama (the practice of breathing), chakra visualization, dance, mindful eating, and many more. These are all valuable and powerful tools, and are essential in your tantric journey. In the previous chapters we have given you detailed guidance on how to integrate these practices into your daily life.

Mastery, however, is something more. It is a level beyond practice. Tantric mastery is not about how long you can hold a breath or how many tantric massage postures you know. No, true tantric mastery is about how you live your life. It's about how you interact with the world around you, how you relate to others and yourself. It's about how you handle your emotions, your desires, your fears. It's about whether you can live in a state of presence, openness and unconditional love, no matter what life throws at you.

As Daniel Odier says in "Tantra: Path of Ecstasy" (1999), "Tantra is not a technique but a love. A love that transcends all conditioning and touches the heart of existence". In other words, the path to tantric mastery is, in essence, a path to love. An all-encompassing love, an all-transforming love. It is not a romantic love, not a platonic love, but a love that is beyond labels and definitions. A love that is born from the center of your being and expands towards infinity, touching and transforming everything in its path.

This kind of love, this kind of mastery, is not something that can be learned in a book or in a class. It is not something that can be measured in hours of practice or skill levels. It is something that is lived, that is experienced, that is embodied.

To help us better understand this concept, let us think of the figure of the Zen master. In Zen, it is said that the true master is not the one who has read all the sacred texts or who can sit in meditation for hours without moving. The true Zen master is one who can see the sacredness in the ordinary, who can find peace in the midst of chaos, who can live in a state of presence and compassion, no matter what the circumstances. As Shunryu Suzuki says in "Zen Mind, Beginner's Mind" (1970), "In the beginner there are many possibilities, in the expert few."

In the same way, the true tantric master is not one who has learned all the techniques and postures, but one who lives from a place of love, presence and openness. One who, in the words of Osho in "Tantra: The Supreme Understanding" (1975), can "transform the mundane into the sacred".

How does one reach that state, how does one move from practice to mastery? Well, the truth is that there is no single answer to these questions. Each of us has our own path, our own experiences, our own learnings. What works for one may not work for another. What takes one person months, another may take years. And that's okay. Tantra, after all, is not a race, but a journey, a process of self-discovery and growth.

However, there are some general principles that can help us on this path. First, it is important to understand that mastery is not a destination, but a path. It is not something that is attained and then maintained, but something that is cultivated and nurtured day by day. In every moment, in every interaction, in every breath, we have the opportunity to practice mastery.

Second, it is important to be patient and kind to yourself. The road to mastery can be long and challenging. There will be moments of doubt, of frustration, of fear. In those moments, it is crucial to remember to be kind to yourself, to remember that every step, no matter how small, is a step in the right direction.

Third, it is essential to maintain an attitude of learning and curiosity. As Jack Kornfield says in "After the Ecstasy, the Laundry" (2000), "The spiritual master is one who keeps learning." In Tantra, as in any other spiritual path, there is always more to learn, more to explore, more to discover. Keeping an open, receptive and curious mind will allow us to keep growing and evolving, no matter how long we have been on the path.

But how does all this apply to the practice of tantric massage? How does one go from performing the movements and techniques to truly embodying the spirit of Tantra? Let's look at a concrete example.

Imagine you are giving a tantric massage to your partner. You've studied the techniques, you've created a sacred space, you've done everything you're supposed to do. And yet, something doesn't feel quite right. Your partner seems to enjoy the massage, but you feel that something is missing, that there is a disconnect between what you are doing and what you are feeling.

At that point, you might panic. You might start judging yourself, questioning your abilities, comparing yourself to others. You might try to force the connection, to do more or do better. But that would only serve to increase disconnection and frustration.

Instead, you could choose to take a deep breath. You could choose to return to your body, to your presence, to your heart. You could choose to remember that you, like your partner, are a sacred being, and that every gesture, every touch, every sigh, is an offering of love.

You could choose, in that instant, to stop doing and start being. To stop acting and start feeling. To stop looking outside and start looking inside.

And in that change of perspective, in that act of surrender and openness, you would find true mastery. Not in the mastery of techniques, but in the recognition of the divinity in yourself and in the other. Not in the perfection of form, but in the authenticity of presence.

This is just one example of how the path to mastery can manifest itself in the practice of tantric massage. There are as many paths as there are people, and each of us will have to discover our own.

So I invite you to take the plunge. To open yourself to the mystery. To allow yourself to be an eternal learner, an eternal seeker. Because, as Rumi says in "The Essential Rumi" (1995), "The seeker is the sought".

Are you ready to embark on this journey? Are you ready to stop being a practitioner and become a master? Are you ready to stop looking outside and start looking inside?

If the answer is yes, then you are ready for the next chapter of your tantric journey. A journey that, as you know, has no end. A journey that is, in itself, the reward.

So, dear reader, get ready for the ecstasy of now. Prepare yourself for a goodbye that is only a new beginning. And always remember that you, like all of us, are a sacred being, a mirror of the divine.

We have already navigated the waves of history and science, danced with the subtleties of energy and desire, explored the corners of our psyche and our heart, and discovered the infinite possibilities that unfold when we dare to surrender to mystery. All this, weaving a path, a tantric path to mastery.

You have faced your fears and resistances, listened to the wisdom of your body and learned to value the power of touch. You have cultivated mindfulness and presence, and discovered the importance of communication and sacred space. You have experienced the pleasure and liberation that integration and transcendence can bring.

Each chapter, each word, each pause, has been a step in this wonderful journey, a milestone on this path of ecstasy. And although this chapter, like the book, comes to an end, the path continues. For the path of Tantra, like the path of life, is a journey without end, an eternal dance of exploration, discovery and surrender.

It is natural to feel a certain melancholy at the end of a book, as it is at the end of any adventure. You may feel nostalgic for the places you've visited, the experiences you've had, the revelations you've had. And that's okay. Melancholy is love's sweet sister, proof that something has touched your heart.

But I also want to invite you to celebrate. To celebrate the road traveled, the challenges overcome, the knowledge acquired.

To celebrate the fact that, even if the book comes to an end, the path of Tantra is still open to you, full of possibilities.

Dear reader, it has been a real pleasure to accompany you on this journey. Your presence, your curiosity, your openness, have made this book possible. Your journey has been my journey, and for that I am deeply grateful.

My wish for you is that you continue exploring, that you continue growing, that you continue awakening. May the light of Tantra illuminate your path and guide you towards fullness, liberation and ecstasy. May you find mastery not only in the practice of tantric massage, but in every aspect of your life.

And always remember that no matter where your journey takes you, you will always be at home in your own body, in your own heart. For you, like all of us, are a sacred being, a mirror of the divine.

With all my love and gratitude, I wish you the best in your tantric path. May every step be a dance, every breath a song, every moment an ecstasy. And may you always, always follow the path of your heart.

Farewell: The Ecstasy of Now: A Farewell Is Only a New Beginning

Here we are, at the end of this fascinating journey through the landscapes of Tantra. It has been an exciting, profound and, I hope, transformative journey. We have delved into the ancient practices of Tantric massage, rediscovering the importance of our five senses and the alchemy of touch, from the skin to the soul. We have learned to breathe life, to awaken the Kundalini energy and to see our body as a temple.

We have faced blockages and resistances, learning to surrender and play with polarity. We have dared to dance with energy and explore the centers of pleasure and energy in our bodies, the chakras. We have integrated meditation and mindfulness into tantric massage, we have discovered the language of the body and healing through touch.

In addition, we have explored different tantric massage techniques and sequences, sought the synthesis of opposites and aspired to transcend time and space. We have reflected on how Tantra can deepen our relationships and how sublimated sexual energy can be channeled into creative power.

Together, we have challenged cultural norms and beliefs and explored the power of sexual energy in both women and men. Finally, we have considered how to achieve enlightenment through pleasure and how to move from practice to mastery on our own path to tantric enlightenment.

As you can see, we have covered a lot of ground. But as with any journey, there is always more to explore. The world of Tantra is vast and deep, and there is always more to learn and experience. So I encourage you to keep exploring, practicing and deepening your understanding and experience of Tantra.

It is my sincere hope that this book has provided you with a useful map for your tantric journey, and that you move forward with courage, curiosity and an open mind. Remember that every step on this path is an act of love for yourself and others, and that the true master of Tantra is none other than your own heart.

With all my love and gratitude for accompanying me on this journey, I wish you the best on your path to tantric mastery. May you always find ecstasy in the now, and may each goodbye be simply a new beginning.

With love, Antonio Jaimez

One last favor

Dear

I hope you enjoyed reading my book. I would like to thank you for taking the time to read it and I hope you found value in its contents. I am writing to you today to make a very important request.

As an independent author, reviews are extremely valuable to me. Not only do they help me get valuable feedback on my work, but they can also influence other readers' decision to buy the book. If you could take a few minutes to leave an honest review on Amazon, it would be a great help to me.

Again, I thank you for taking the time to read my book and for considering my review request. Your feedback and support means a lot to me as an independent author.

You can also find more books on this subject from my Amazon author page.

https://www.amazon.es/~/e/B0C4TS75MD

You can also visit my website <u>www.libreriaonlinemax.com</u> where you will find all kinds of hypnosis explained in detail, hypnotherapies, free resources and expert level courses. You can also use the following QR code:

Best regards,

Antonio Jaimez

Printed in Great Britain
by Amazon

38698089R00106